Vitamins & Minerals

Graham Yost

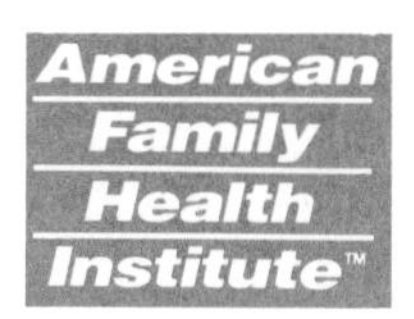

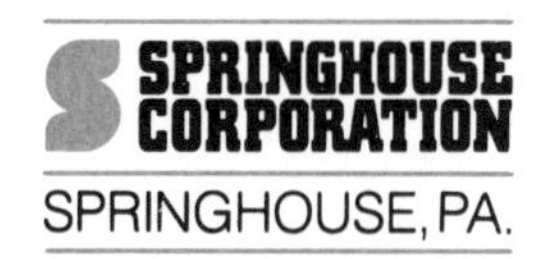

SPRINGHOUSE, PA.

Program Director
Stanley Loeb

Clinical Director
Barbara McVan, RN

Art Director
John Hubbard

Editors
Nancy Priff
Kevin Law
Beth Mauro
June Norris

Designer
Maria Errico

Editorial Services Supervisor
David Moreau

Production Manager
Wilbur Davidson

The charter of the American Family Health Institute is to research and produce high-quality publications that enhance the health of individuals and their families. Essential to health are physical, emotional, and social well-being, not just the absence of illness or infirmity. The Institute's Medical Board has produced the *Health and Fitness* books to share up-to-date and authoritative information that can give readers greater personal control over their health maintenance.

Library of Congress Cataloging-in-Publication Data
Yost, Graham.
Vitamins and minerals.
(Health and fitness series)
Includes index.
1. Vitamins in human nutrition. 2. Minerals in human nutrition. I. Brunner, Lillian Sholtis. II. American Family Health Institute. Medical Board. III. Title. IV. Series. Health and fitness series. [DNLM: 1. Minerals—popular works. 2. Vitamins—popular works. QU 160 Y65v]
QP771.Y67 1986 613.2'8 85-30279
ISBN 0-87434-020-9

The procedures and explanations given in this publication are based on research and consultation with medical and nursing authorities. To the best of our knowledge, these procedures and explanations reflect currently accepted medical practice; nevertheless, they can't be considered absolute and universal recommendations. For individual application, treatment suggestions must be considered in light of the individual's health, subject to a doctor's specific recommendations. The authors and the publisher disclaim responsibility for any adverse effects resulting directly or indirectly from the suggested procedures, from any undetected errors, or from the reader's misunderstanding of the text.

Contents

Vitamins & Minerals

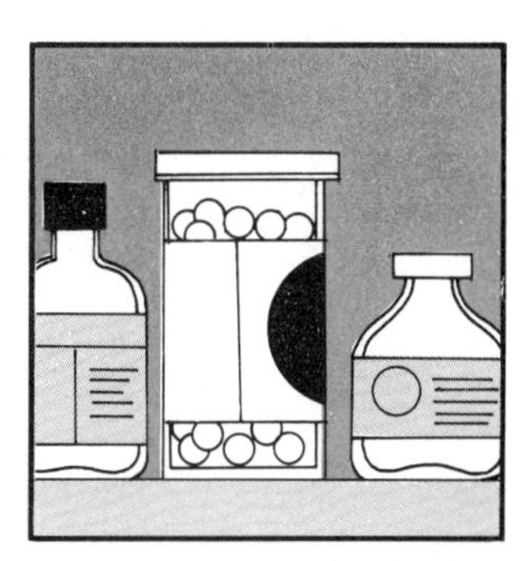

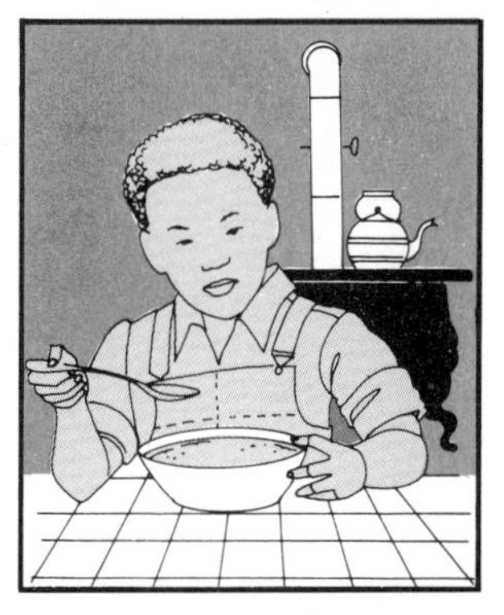

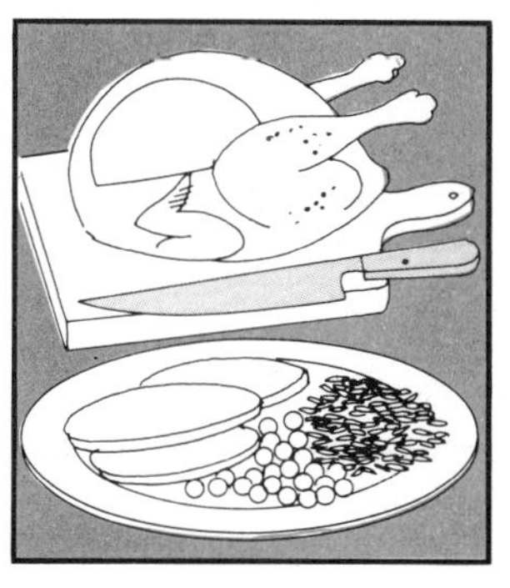

1

Vitamins & minerals: new kids on the block

Important discoveries
Until vitamins and minerals were discovered, no one knew why the food people eat is directly related to health. People saw nothing wrong with eating a steady diet of the same foods. Even when people discovered that certain foods help in the treatment of certain diseases, they didn't know that the answer lay in vitamins.

Zoe is a sailor with His Majesty's navy. It's a dangerous time for sailors—a time when the greatest threat comes not from pirates or Spanish galleons, but from "the *scurvy*," a dread disease that can be counted on to claim the lives of up to half the men on any voyage. Like others on board, Zoe eats a diet of salted meat, biscuits, and dried beans. And like many of the others, his breath turns horribly foul, his gums bleed, his legs stop working, and his teeth fall out. Zoe's put ashore to die. Unable to move, he stuffs some grass in his mouth, and after a few days of eating just that he finds, to his surprise, he has the strength to walk again. He's picked up by a passing ship, and his story of how what he ate cured his scurvy travels fast.

Scurvy had been the scourge of sailors for 200 years, and when British naval physician James Lind heard Zoe's tale, he set out to find what foods could stop the disease. His *Treatise on Scurvy* described how he reversed and prevented the disorder in British sailors by giving them lime juice. (This is the basis for the nickname *limeys*.) In 1795, a year after his death, Lind's prescription of lemons was followed by the British navy, and scurvy ceased to plague British sailors. It wasn't until 1928, however, that the anti-scurvy factor in citrus fruits was isolated. We now know it as *Vitamin C*.

The pellagra preventive

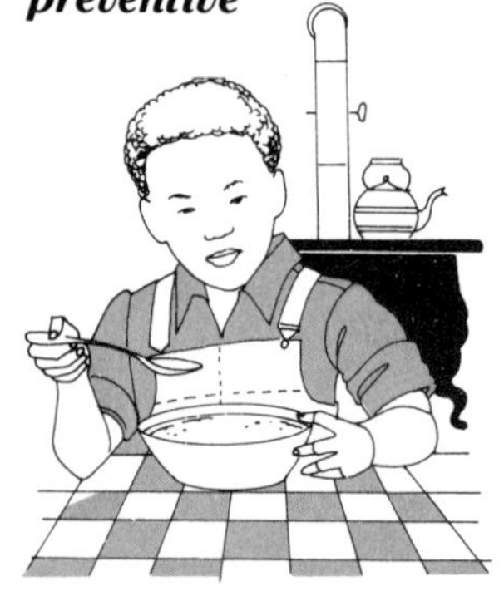

Dr. Joseph Goldberger discovered that pellagra was caused by a vitamin deficiency. Goldberger made the discovery in 1915, and he called his discovery "the pellagra preventive." Today we know it as niacin, or Vitamin B_3.

The American South, early 1900s
Corn's about all Jack's family can afford, so it's about all they eat. Cornmeal mush, day in, day out, with maybe a strip of salted fat or a bit of blackstrap molasses thrown in as a treat. And Jack, like the rest of his family, doesn't feel too well. His bones ache, and it's hard to think straight. His Dad's worse—he gets truly crazy sometimes, and there doesn't seem to be anything anyone can do about it.

There was something they could have done about it, but no one knew it then. Jack's family had *pellagra*, a disease common among poor people throughout the South in the early 1900s. Like scurvy, it's a deficiency

Taking away the sun

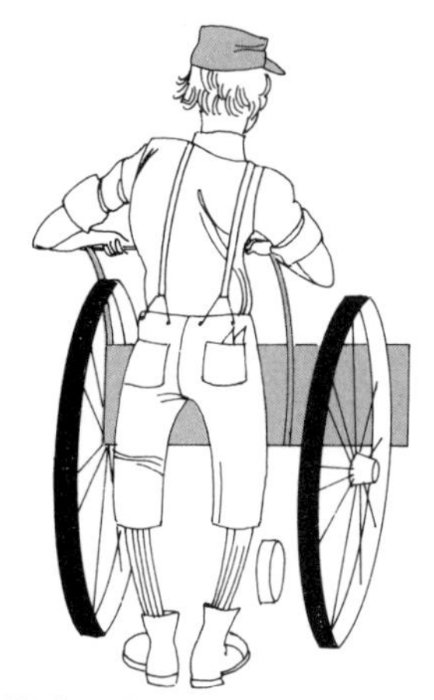

Rickets became common in Europe during the Industrial Revolution, when people spent the daylight hours working indoors seven days a week. Many workers went to work before sun up and returned home after dark. The lack of sunlight—and Vitamin D—caused rickets.

"I cannot"

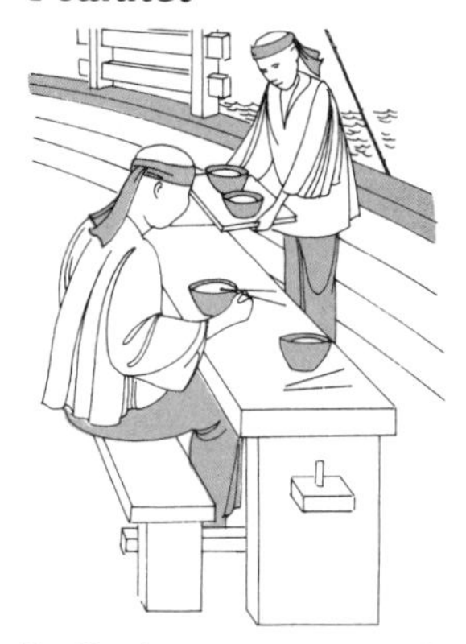

Beriberi was a common disease throughout the Orient during the 1800s. Its name comes from the language of Ceylon and means "I cannot"—an indication of the weakness and degeneration that characterize the disease.

disease, brought about by a lack of *Vitamin* B_3—niacin—in the diet. It took a while to track this down, but when the cure was found, and foods rich in the vitamin—milk, eggs, vegetables, and meat—were added to the all-corn diet, families like Jack's sprang back to health within days.

Industrial England, 1800s

Archie's only 12, but he works in a Birmingham factory 14 hours a day, six or seven days a week, and has done so for as long as he can remember. About all he sees of the sun are a few stray rays filtered through a sooty window high in the factory wall. And Archie's in pain. His elbows and knees ache, his legs are bowed as if he'd been riding a horse all his life, and his spine's starting to hunch up.

He's got *rickets*. And while the medical profession of the day searched in vain for a rickets-causing germ, the true cure was simple: give the sufferers some time in the sun and a spoonful of cod-liver oil. Archie and other rickets sufferers were deficient in *Vitamin D*, a vitamin we get from sunlight and certain foods, crucial in keeping our bones straight and strong.

The Japanese navy, 1882

Toshiro is a sailor, and what he fears most are not sharks or typhoons, but the lethal *beriberi*, which starts by making men sway as they walk, then leads to paralysis, insanity, and death. Toshiro would be lucky if he didn't get it. In 1882, over 41 percent of the Japanese navy was lost to its ravages—a total of almost 2,000 men. But if Toshiro makes it through that year and the next four after that, he'll be home free because beriberi will no longer be a threat.

Before 1884, Japanese sailors subsisted on a diet of polished rice—rice with the husks removed. But in 1884, when they were put on a new diet that included vegetables, oats, and milk, the beriberi disappeared. For years, scientists searched for something in the polished rice that caused the disease and found nothing. Eventually, they discovered it was something *missing* from polished rice that did it, for by polishing the rice—removing the rice husks—people were also removing *Vitamin* B_1—*thiamine*.

The discovery of vitamins

Scurvy, pellagra, rickets, and beriberi are the four most notorious vitamin deficiency ailments. When scientists discovered what caused these illnesses, they also discovered vitamins—but not without some resistance. The big thing in science and medicine in the 1800s was infection. Wherever there was an illness, scientists went searching for the germ causing it, vehemently rejecting the idea that a cure could be anything as simple as something in food (in earlier days, scientists pooh-poohed germs, scoffing at the idea that things they couldn't see—germs—could cause so much trouble).

A few vitamin pioneers stuck to their guns. One of them was Casimir Funk, who, in the early part of this century, discovered both thiamine and niacin. He also coined the phrase *vitamine*—*vita* meaning "life" in Latin, and an *amine* being an organic compound with nitrogen in it (when it was found that not all these substances were amines, the "e" was dropped, and they became just vitamins).

What is malnutrition?

Malnutrition includes any nutritional disorder, whether from an unbalanced, insufficient, or excessive diet or because of poor absorption, assimilation, or use of foods by the body. Although it's most common in underdeveloped nations, malnutrition also occurs in industrialized countries.

No matter what the cause, the effects of malnutrition can be severe. It can produce muscle wasting, apathy, loss of appetite, lethargy, weakness, and susceptibility to infections, as well as the signs you see here.

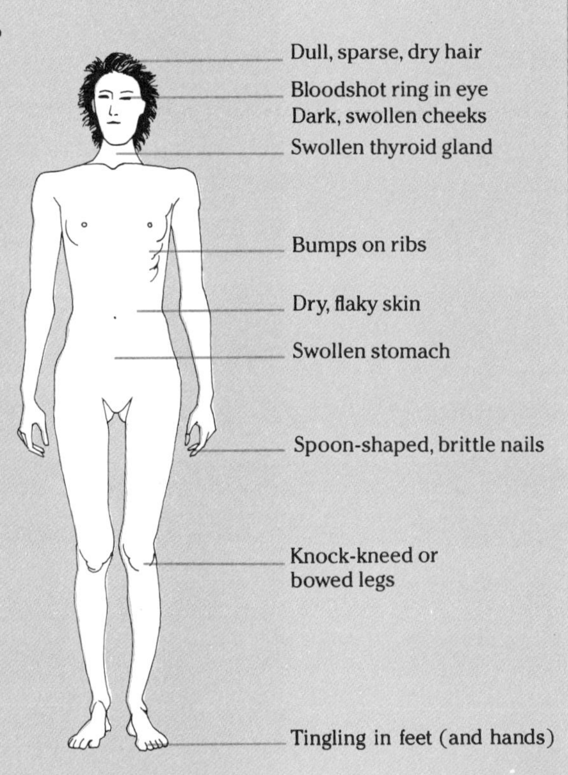

Vitamins weren't the only things scoffed at. For a long time no one would believe that the same minerals mined from the earth could also play an important role in the human body. We now know that mineral deficiencies can cause trouble (as examples, lack of iron can lead to anemia, a condition that leaves you weak and tired; low calcium, osteoporosis, an affliction that makes your bones brittle and easy to break), yet not until the 1940s were such minerals treated with due regard.

The days of such gross and widespread deficiencies as pellagra are thankfully long gone in our country (although not around the world). But just because you'll never have to worry about beriberi doesn't mean you shouldn't think about vitamins and minerals. They do a lot more than cure scurvy and rickets, and it's good to have an idea of what they do and how they do it.

The incredible human machine

You may have heard some astounding claims over the past few years concerning the ability of vitamins and minerals to do this or that for you. You may have heard people say that vitamins can cure everything from cancer to the common cold, from baldness to sexual disorders. Many of these claims are absurdly outlandish, but others seem more reasonable. What should you believe? While only a few vitamins and minerals are harmful, and even then only in high doses, you should still wait until more of the reports are in before you start wolfing down handfuls of Vitamin A to correct your nearsightedness. However, whether or not vitamins and minerals turn out to be the wonder potions some people think they are, what we already know about them shows them to be really quite amazing.

Treating vitamins and minerals sensibly

Vitamins and minerals are vital to life and perform a wide range of functions in our bodies. Don't underestimate their importance, but don't overestimate it, either. Remember these basic guidelines:

- *Vitamin and mineral supplements aren't substitutes for a balanced diet.*
- *If your daily diet includes foods from the major food groups, you won't have vitamin or mineral deficiencies.*
- *Vitamin and mineral supplements are drugs and should be respected as such. Don't take overdoses of these drugs, and don't leave them within reach of children.*

Think of this: a serious deficiency in only one vitamin can bring about disastrous physical consequences in weeks or even days. In fact, you simply cannot live without a full complement of vitamins and minerals. But that's not really as scary as it sounds, because about the only place you could ever completely remove a vitamin from a person's diet would be in a laboratory. That's because they're in just about everything you eat (although in varying amounts).

To get an idea of how the vitamins on your plate keep the incredible human machine running, we should first look at how that machine uses food—its fuel.

Digestion

Digestion is the process by which your body breaks food down into simpler elements so that these elements can be absorbed into the bloodstream and used for energy, repair of tissues, and growth. The digestive process begins the moment you put a forkful of food in your mouth. As your teeth grind and cut up the food, it's mixed with saliva, beginning a process of breaking it down chemically. When you swallow, you start the mechanism that pushes and kneads the food along the digestive tract.

The first stop is the stomach, where the food is churned and mixed with highly acidic gastric juices that further break down what you've eaten. But while we often think of the stomach as where we digest food, that's not really the case. First, a matter of geography—your stomach's located just under your lower ribs (when you hear your "stomach" rumble, it's actually your lower intestine that's making the noise). Also, food isn't completely digested in your stomach, just broken down and prepared for absorption (about the only thing absorbed into your blood through your stomach is alcohol). In fact, the stomach isn't necessary for life. People who've had their stomachs removed for medical reasons have survived quite well.

Absorption of food really occurs in the small intestine, which really isn't very small at all—it's about 23 feet long. As food is pushed out of the stomach and into the small intestine, it's mixed with bile and fatty

The digestive tract

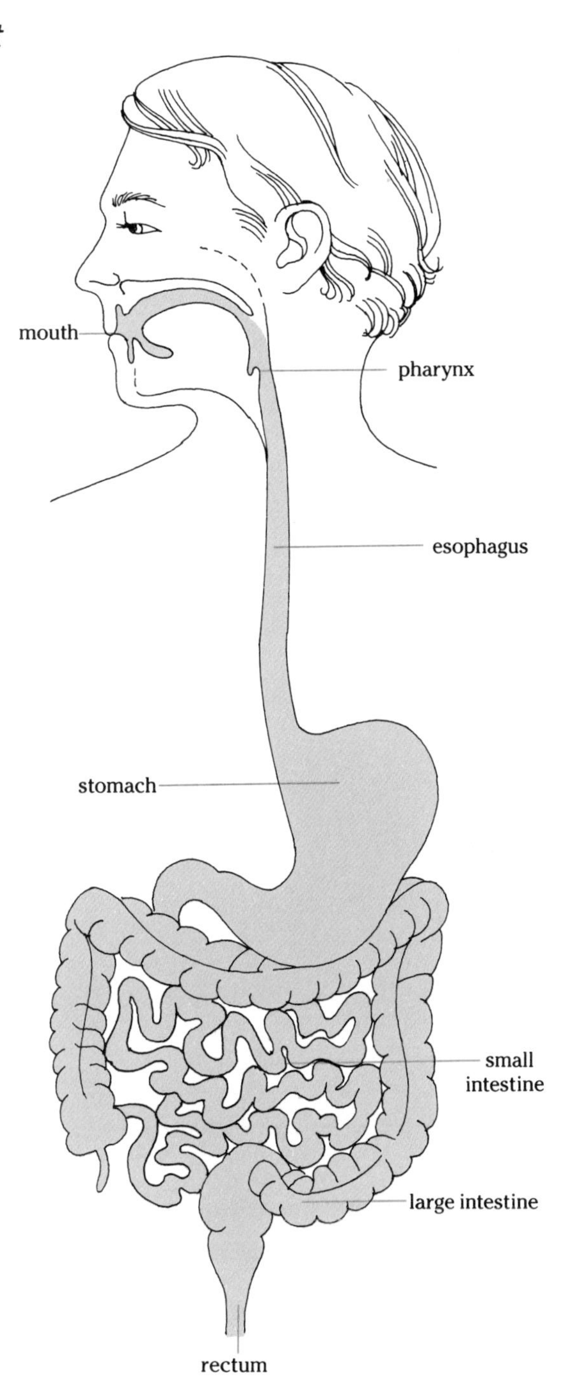

Digestion takes place in the digestive tract, or alimentary canal. In the mouth, teeth grind and cut up food, and the food is mixed with saliva, beginning the process of breaking it down chemically. The food next passes through the pharynx and esophagus into the stomach, where the food is churned and mixed with gastric juices that break it down further. The food then passes into the small intestine, from which it is absorbed; the large intestine (colon); and it then leaves the body through the rectum as waste. The entire alimentary canal is about 30 feet long.

acids, and the nutrients that the body wants are absorbed through the intestine wall and taken into the bloodstream. When all the good has been taken out of the food, what's left, waste product, is passed along into the large intestine (colon) and eventually out of the body. It takes about 20 hours for your body to process a forkful of food.

The chemicals that do the digesting are manufactured by three vital organs in your body: the liver, gallbladder, and pancreas.

The *liver* weighs about four pounds and is your largest internal organ. It's a fantastic chemical plant that we still do not understand entirely. We know it manufactures several key items; stores Vitamin A, and glycogen (an energy reserve); and works as a processing plant, rendering toxic substances safe. The liver is important to digestion because it produces bile. Bile excreted by your liver is held by your *gallbladder,* where the bile is concentrated before being sent into your small intestine to act on incoming food.

The *pancreas* is the third organ involved. Part of it manufactures insulin, the chemical that regulates how

Organs that aid digestion

The liver, gallbladder, and pancreas manufacture chemicals for the digestion process. The liver is located on the right side of the abdominal cavity just under the diaphragm. A pear-shaped sac, the gallbladder is located just under the liver. The pancreas, about 6 inches long, is located across and behind the stomach.

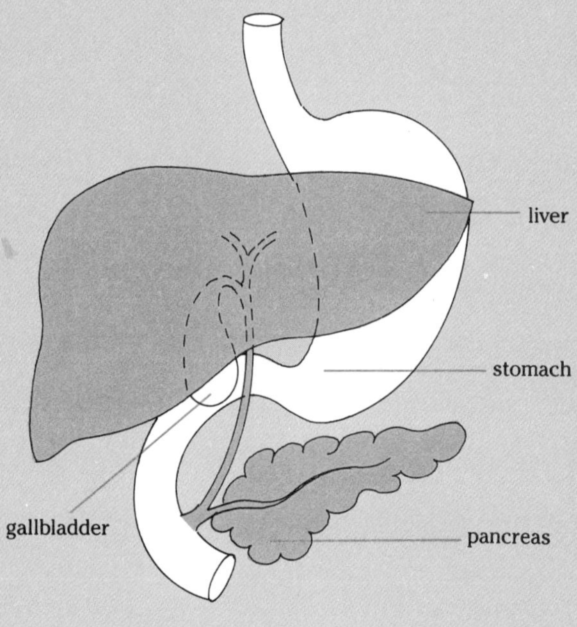

sugar is burned in your blood. The pancreas also produces pancreatic juice, containing some of your body's most crucial enzymes, needed to split fats, proteins, and starches. Together, the liver, gallbladder, and pancreas help get nutrients out of food, through the walls of your digestive tract, and into your bloodstream where they can go to work.

Size isn't everything
Even though they're called macro *("big") and* micro *("small") nutrients, both are equally important in fueling your body and keeping it running well.*

Macronutrients
Oxygen
Water
Protein
Carbohydrates
Fats

Micronutrients
Vitamins
Minerals

Nutrients: keeping the machine in working order

The nutrients that keep your body working properly are divided into two groups: *macronutrients* and *micronutrients*. Macronutrients, as their name suggests, are big nutrients, raw material for your body. They're oxygen, water, proteins, carbohydrates, and fats.

Oxygen

Oxygen's easy to overlook as a nutrient, maybe because we're breathing all the time and take it for granted, but also because there doesn't seem to be anything solid or substantial about it. In the human machine it's vital, for your body can burn fuel only when it's combined with oxygen, and if the supply of oxygen is cut off you'll die.

Water

Water can also be overlooked as a nutrient because it too doesn't seem to have any value of its own. But not only is water what helps regulate your body temperature; it's also what you're mostly made of (up to 75 percent). Just as much as they need oxygen, our bodies depend on water—you can survive for weeks without food, but a few days without water and you could be in serious trouble.

Proteins

Your body uses proteins for cell building, growth, and internal repair. Proteins provide the building material for the muscles, blood, skin, hair, nails, and the internal organs. Your body also needs protein to form hormones, enzymes, and antibodies. However, it only needs a certain amount of protein (about a third of a gram for every pound of body weight), and any excess is either burned off or converted to fat.

Amino acids
When food is digested, the protein in it is broken down into amino acids. Your body then puts these amino acids together again in various combinations to make the kinds of protein required by the muscles, red blood cells, and other body tissue; any remaining amino acids are broken down further to supply energy.

Proteins are made of a variety of amino acids, which are vital for proper growth, development, and health. The body can form 14 (nonessential) amino acids, but it has to get 8 others (essential) from foods. When a food has all 8 essential amino acids, it's called a *com-*

Metabolism
Metabolism is the body's biochemical processes that build up living tissue from basic food materials or breaks down food to provide energy. Protein, carbohydrates, and fats are ***metabolized*** *to produce new tissue and to produce energy.*

plete protein. Complete proteins include meat, poultry, fish, eggs, milk, and cheese. When a food lacks the 8 essential amino acids, it's an *incomplete* protein. Some examples are nuts, navy beans, and chick peas.

Carbohydrates

Carbohydrates are the energy sources that your body burns to keep running. The digestive process breaks them down into sugars; then the liver turns them into glucose. Glucose is then either used as fuel, or, if there's extra, stored in your liver and muscles as glycogen, an energy reserve. Once your liver and muscles have what they need, leftover glucose is stored as fat. When you exercise, you first burn off the glucose just produced by your liver, then the reserve glycogen. Once those are gone you start on the fats, and when they're depleted (in endurance sports or on starvation diets), your body has to start burning proteins.

Fats

Fat is not only your body's most efficient energy reserve, it also plays a key role in your metabolism in the form of fatty acids. Not only are they involved in the construction of cells, hormones, and some body fluids, but fatty acids are needed for the fat-soluble vitamins A, D, E, and K to be absorbed and transported.

Those are the macronutrients: oxygen, water, proteins, carbohydrates, and fats. They're the big things you take into your body in bulk—so big that you can actually see some of them. You breathe oxygen as you inhale. You drink water directly, but you also get it from

Fat soluble, water soluble: what does it mean?

Fat-soluble vitamins require the presence of fats or oils in your digestive tract to be absorbed into your body. They often can be found in the fatty portions of food (not just meat—they appear in fruits and vegetables as well). The other characteristic about fat-soluble vitamins is that they can be stored in your liver and other organs and tissues. Water-soluble vitamins require water in your digestive tract to be absorbed into your body. They aren't stored in significant amounts by your body and must be replaced daily.

Fat soluble	***Water soluble***	
Vitamin A	*Thiamine*	*Biotin*
Vitamin D	*Riboflavin*	*Folic acid*
Vitamin E	*Niacin*	*Pantothenate*
Vitamin K	*Pyridoxine*	*Vitamin C*

fruits, vegetables, and other liquids. When you eat meat you get protein. You eat some potatoes, you get some carbohydrates. You eat peanut butter or ice cream, and you get some fats. But mixed in with these macronutrients, in tiny amounts you can't taste and could see only with a microscope, are the micronutrients. And small as they are, without micronutrients—vitamins and minerals—the machine would come to a halt.

Vitamins and minerals: what they are and what they do

Vitamins are organic compounds essential to life. Each vitamin is a specific grouping of elements responsible for regulating your vital metabolic processes. There are two kinds of vitamins: fat soluble, which dissolve in fats and oils, and water soluble, which dissolve in water.

For the mere handful of vitamins we know of, there are an extraordinary number of names. Most have a letter name (such as A, B, C) as well as several chemical word names (such as ascorbic acid, thiamine, niacin.) To make matters more confusing, after they had been given letter names, it was discovered that Vitamin B was in fact several different vitamins, all chemically distinct, each with its own job to do, and so they became known as the B-complex vitamins (B_1, B_2, B_6, and so on).

Here's a quick look at each of the vitamins and the role it performs.

Vitamin A

A fat-soluble vitamin. Like all fat solubles it requires fatty acids to absorb it through the digestive tract. It's stored in your liver. It comes primarily in two forms, one from animal products, the other from both animals and plants. Vitamin A is a key ingredient in the pigment in your eyes that allows you to see in dim light, so a deficiency in it can lead to night blindness.

Vitamin B_1 (Thiamine hydrocloride)

Like all B-complex vitamins it's water soluble, which means it doesn't get stored in the body and must be replaced daily. B_1 and all B-complex vitamins work better as a family than they do alone (the old maxim: the whole is greater than the sum of the parts). B_1 is vital in turning your body's fuel—carbohydrates—into energy.

Working synergistically

The B-complex vitamins work synergistically—the total effect of the B-complex vitamins taken together is greater than the effect of the vitamins taken separately. Simply, each B-complex vitamin can do more for you if you take it with the other members of the B-complex family.

Vitamin B_2 (Riboflavin)
Water soluble; this vitamin must be replaced daily. Your cells need B_2 to help them get oxygen and get rid of carbon dioxide. One key characteristic of B_2 is that it doesn't survive exposure to sunlight for long, which is why it's better to keep milk in an opaque container like a carton rather than a plastic or glass jug.

Niacin (Vitamin B_3, nicotinic acid)
Water soluble; this vitamin must be replaced daily. This is one of the few vitamins the body can produce itself, but only if a certain amino acid and several other B-complex vitamins are present. A very important vitamin, it helps your cells breathe and use other nutrients.

Vitamin B_6 (Pyridoxine hydrochloride)
Water soluble; this vitamin must be replaced daily. It assembles the amino acids that make up proteins that in turn are used to make cells.

Vitamin B_{12} (Cyanocobalamin)
Water soluble; this vitamin must be replaced daily. It plays a key role in regulating your nervous system functions.

How the body absorbs Vitamin B_{12}

1. Person eats food containing Vitamin B_{12}.
2. In the stomach, B_{12} forms a complex with intrinsic factor—a substance found in the body.
3. B_{12} complex travels to special sites in the small intestine, where it's absorbed.
4. B_{12} separates from the intrinsic factor.
5. B_{12} enters the bloodstream to travel to body tissues.
6. Body excretes some excess B_{12} in urine.
7. Liver stores some excess B_{12}.

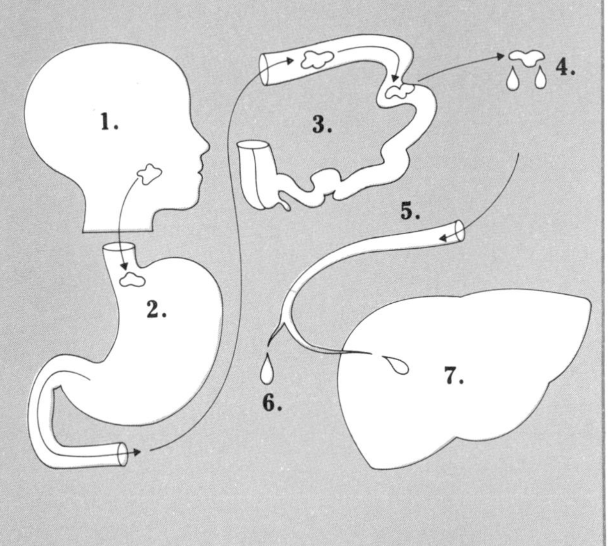

You and the bulbul bird

Most animals produce their own Vitamin C, but humans don't—nor, for that matter, do monkeys, guinea pigs, the bulbul bird, and a certain fruit-eating bat in India.

Vitamin F?

Some substances that many don't consider vitamins have vitamin names. Vitamin F *is the name sometimes given to essential fatty acids.* Vitamin P *is what some call the bioflavonoids, substances that accompany* Vitamin C *in citrus foods and that may make it more effective.*

Biotin

A fairly recent discovery in the B-complex family, and like other Bs it's water soluble and must be replaced every day. Biotin is still something of a mystery, although its importance to the thyroid and adrenal glands and in many metabolic and enzyme reactions is known.

Folic acid (Folate, Vitamin B_9, Folacin)

Another recently discovered B-complex family member. Water soluble; this vitamin must be replaced daily. Its function in metabolism is still something of a mystery. It does play an important role in cell division and reproduction.

Pantothenate (Pantothenic acid, Panthenol)

Another not yet fully understood B vitamin, again water soluble and requiring daily replacement. It works with the adrenal glands and may have something to do with how your body deals with stress.

Vitamin C (Ascorbic acid)

Water soluble; this vitamin must be replaced daily. Any excess Vitamin C is flushed out of your body in a few hours. Vitamin C is vital for the growth, strength, and health of most tissues in your body. Key attributes: it keeps your blood vessels strong and helps keep your blood from clotting in your veins.

Vitamin D

A fat-soluble vitamin that you produce all by yourself, just by exposing your skin to sunlight. When ultraviolet light hits your skin, the oils present produce the vitamin, which is then absorbed through the skin. Vitamin D is essential in helping the minerals calcium and phosphorus build cartilage and bone.

Vitamin E

A fat-soluble vitamin, stored in the liver, other internal organs, and the blood. Unlike other fat solubles, it doesn't stay stored for long and needs more regular replacement. Key attribute: E stops the essential fatty acids in us from oxidizing (combining with oxygen and spoiling). Like Vitamin C, E also helps prevent blood from clotting in your veins.

Is it a vitamin?

Vitamins are organic compounds essential to life. With few exceptions, they can't be made by the body and must be gotten from food or vitamin supplements. The body must have vitamins in small amounts to regulate its normal processes, or metabolism.

If a researcher finds a new substance that meets these criteria, it could be a vitamin.

Vitamin K

A fat-soluble vitamin that, for the most part, your body synthesizes from its own internal bacteria. It gets its name from a Scandinavian word, *koagulation*, which, like the English *coagulation*, means the clotting of blood. Vitamin K is essential—without it, a cut finger wouldn't stop bleeding because the blood wouldn't clot. Newborn babies haven't yet started to produce it, so one of the first things they get is a shot of Vitamin K.

Other vitamins

Several substances may or may not turn out to be vitamins. They have some vitamin characteristics but have yet to be shown to be either essential or to be true vitamins. *Choline* is an example. It's found with a number of B-complex vitamins and may have something to do with breaking down fats and cholesterol. On the other hand, it's found in such high quantities in your body that it may be a structural component rather than a metabolic regulator like a vitamin. *Inositol* is another questionable substance associated with the B complex. What it does is unclear, although it too may reduce cholesterol buildup. *PABA (para-aminobenzoic acid)* is also associated with B-complex vitamins. Not a lot is known about it except that when used in an ointment it makes an effective sunscreen.

Then there are the extremely controversial "vitamins" *orotic acid* (B_{13}), *pangamic acid* (B_{15}), *Laetrile* (B_{17}), *Vitamin Q*, *Vitamin U*, and *Vitamin T*. There's not much reliable information on any of them. Russian scientists say pangamic acid can cure hangovers; Vitamin U, a raw cabbage extract, is said to cure stomach ulcers; Laetrile, an extract of apricot pits, is said to cure cancer. In fact, Vitamin Q is the only one about which extravagant claims are not made. It was discovered by Dr. Armand J. Quick who found it helpful in treating a rare hereditary bleeding disorder and doesn't claim it can do any more than that.

Scientists aren't finished adding to the list of vitamins. New substances are discovered every year, and while they're often just old vitamins seen in a new light, doing a new job, or are compounds of questionable merit, a Vitamin X or a Vitamin Z may be waiting to be found.

A vitamin by any other name...

Not only do all the vitamins have letter and word names, they can also have a variety of different word names. Some of the names listed below are for chemically different forms of the vitamin (carotene and retinol are two different forms of Vitamin A), but many are simply separate names that have clung to these substances over the years.

Vitamin	Other names*
Vitamin A	Retinol; dehydroretinol; retinaldehyde; retinoic acid; alpha-, beta-, or gamma-carotene; carotin; provitamin A
Vitamin D	Cholecalciferol, ergocalciferol, calciferon, ergosterol, Vitamin D_2, Vitamin D_3, sunshine vitamin
Vitamin E	Alpha-tocopherol
Vitamin K	Phytonadione, menaquinone, menadione, menadiol, phylloquinone
Vitamin C	Ascorbic acid, rose hips, the antiscorbutic vitamin
Thiamine	Vitamin B_1
Riboflavin	Vitamin B_2, Vitamin G
Niacin	Niacinanide, nicotinic acid, nicotinamide, Vitamin B_3
Vitamin B_6	Pyridoxine, pyridoxal, pyridoxamine, pyrodoxine hydrochloride
Folic acid	Folacin, Vitamin M, Vitamin B_9, pteroylglutamic acid, pteroylmonoglutamic acid, pteroic acid, folate, folinic acid
Vitamin B_{12}	Cobalamin, Castle's extrinsic factor, hydroxocobalamin, cyanocobalamin
Pantothenic acid	Panthenol, pantothenol, calcium pantothenate, pantothen
Biotin	Vitamin H

*These include chemically distinct forms of some vitamins.

Working together

Calcium is an example of a mineral that can't do its job without the presence of a certain vitamin. Calcium can't be absorbed without Vitamin D. That's one reason why Vitamin D has been added to milk.

Minerals

Minerals are the other class of micronutrients found in food. The minerals in food come in very small quantities, just like vitamins. A strong relationship exists between these two micronutrients; some vitamins can't do their jobs without certain minerals being present, and vice versa.

The difference between vitamins and minerals is that while vitamins are organic compounds of elements (perhaps carbon and nitrogen with silicon), minerals are the irreducible elements themselves. Also, while the body can produce some vitamins itself, it can't produce a single mineral. There's another difference—minerals don't have a lot of different letters, numbers, and names. They're called by the same names we learned in chemistry class, for the iron in a nail is basically the same as the iron in a leaf of spinach.

Here's a quick look at the essential minerals in food:

Calcium

A key ingredient in the plaster casts used to set broken bones, it's also a key ingredient in the bones themselves. There are about three pounds of this mineral in your body, making it a *bulk mineral*. Ninety-nine percent of it goes into your bones and teeth, making them strong and hard, and the remaining 1 percent can be found in your body's fluids and tissues. Without calcium in your blood, you'd have convulsions.

Chromium

The mineral that's used to make chrome is the same mineral your body uses to help insulin do its job of burning sugar in the bloodstream (although in a different, nontoxic form, so don't go chewing on a bumper to get your chromium). But while with calcium we speak of amounts the size of grams and kilograms present in the body, with chromium, there are only a few hundred *micrograms* (mcg.)—one one-millionth of a gram—around. Therefore, chromium is known as a *trace mineral*.

Copper

Also a trace mineral, copper is involved in everything from your ability to absorb and use iron in your blood to your sense of taste.

Fluorine

For decades it's been added to our water supply in an effort to reduce tooth decay, and that it does (although in too great amounts it will actually discolor teeth). It may also prevent bone loss.

Iodine

A trace mineral. Iodine is crucial to the formation of a hormone in the thyroid gland, which in turn regulates the metabolic rate of your body. (See Understanding iodine and goiter, page 20.)

Iron

The most important trace mineral. Over 70 percent of the body's iron combines with protein to form hemoglobin, the part of your blood that carries oxygen. The liver, spleen, and bone store most of the rest. The body uses only as much iron as it needs. (Any dietary excess is excreted in the feces.) As red blood cells die, the body recycles the iron in the hemoglobin, instead of excreting it.

Calcium's role in bone formation

More than 90% of the body's calcium is stored in the skeleton, where the bones are constantly being eroded and built up. As you'll see, calcium plays a major part in the buildup of bone. Here's how:

The periosteum—a layer of dense connective tissue—surrounds the bone, which is made of columns of calcified tissue. Each column, or Haversian system, is filled with fluid and contains an artery, vein, and lymph vessels. Bone forms when osteoblasts—bone-forming cells—lay down rings of calcium, phosphorus, and other minerals in the framework of the cartilage.

In some bones, collagen fibers run between the layers of calcium and minerals for extra strength. In other bones, the columns are loosely packed and the collagen forms a honeycomb pattern for lightness.

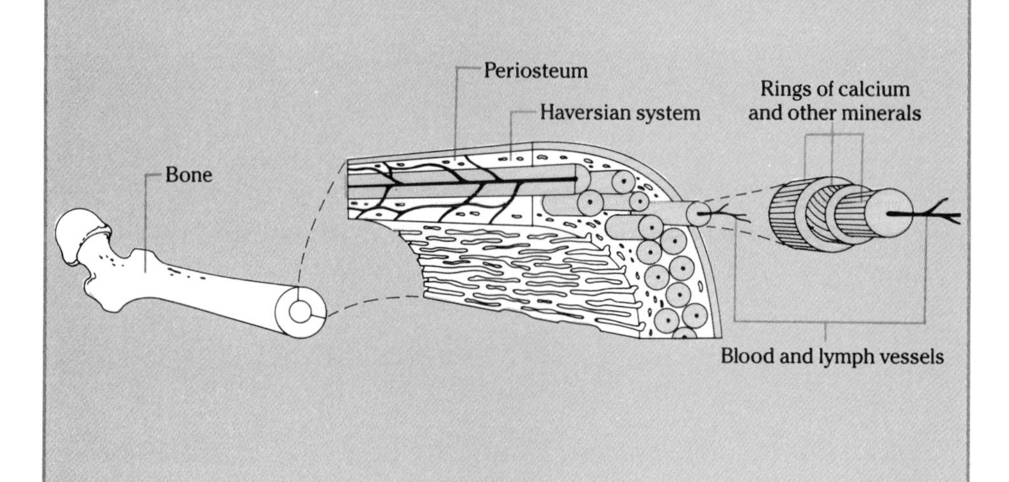

Magnesium
There's not a lot of magnesium in your body (0.05 percent of your total body weight), but enough that it's considered more than a trace mineral. More than half of it is found in the bone. It's involved in regulating cell metabolism and growth.

Manganese
A trace mineral. It works with proteins in the formation of cartilage and is involved with the acids that make up your cells' genetic coding. It also helps insulin do its job and may play a part in breaking down fats.

Phosphorus
After calcium, phosphorus is the second most prevalent mineral in your body and is plentiful in most foods. Its major role is its teamwork with calcium in making bones and teeth strong. It can also be found in every cell of your body, taking part in almost every metabolic process.

Understanding iodine and goiter

Iodine is found in all cells, but its main job is in the thyroid gland, where it helps form the hormone thyroxine. When the thyroid gland doesn't get enough iodine, it enlarges to try to overcome the deficiency. The enlarged gland is known as a goiter. Because of their hormonal link, iodine deficiency and goiter are more common in women, especially during menarche (the first menstruation), pregnancy, and menopause.

Typically, iodine exists in the soil and in things that grow in the soil. But in certain parts of the world, iodine-poor soil produces iodine-poor food, and the people who eat it are likely to develop a goiter, unless they supplement their diet with iodine somehow.

In the United States, the "goiter belt" includes Nebraska, North and South Dakota, the Great Lakes area, Colorado, Montana, Utah, Oregon, and Washington. The map here shows other parts of the world where iodine deficiency and goiter are common.

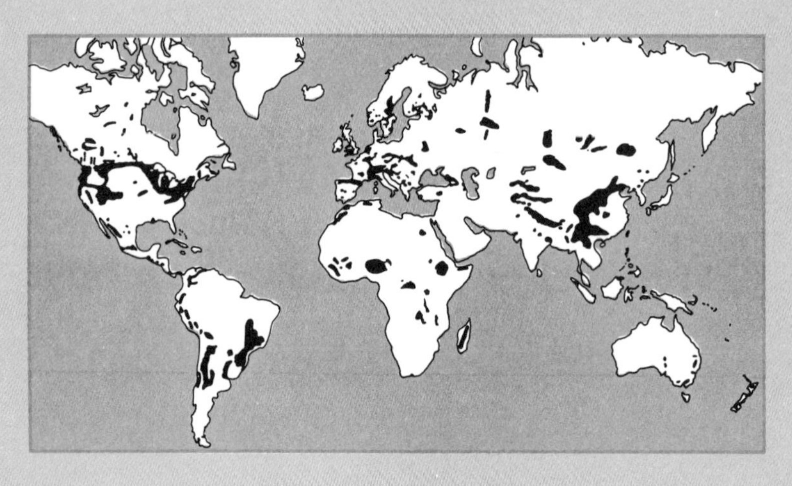

Potassium
The third most prevalent mineral. You've got about nine ounces of it inside you at any time. It's involved in enzyme reactions, in how your nerves react, and in how your muscles work (which is why athletes are always worrying about keeping their potassium intake high).

Selenium
Like all trace minerals, too much selenium can be harmful, and for a long time it was looked at as a poison. Now it's seen as Vitamin E's best partner, helping E do its work. There's also some indication it might be useful in combating heart disease and cancer.

Silicon
A trace mineral. Made out of the same thing glass and computer chips are—sand. Helps keep your bones and connective tissues healthy.

Sodium
We get a lot of this one, probably too much, in the form of salt. It's still important, though, keeping fluids and nutrients moving in and out of your cells. It too is a bulk mineral.

Zinc
After iron, the second most important trace mineral, involved in cell growth, dozens of enzyme reactions, the flushing of carbon dioxide from the cells, and much more.

How vitamins measure up

International units? Grams? Micrograms? What are these measurements? Although they're all units of measure for vitamins and minerals, they're very different. Here are some of the common metric measurements that you can expect to see:

- *Gram (gm)—a unit of weight that equals .03 ounce (1 gm = .03 oz.)*
- *Milligram (mg)—a unit of weight that equals one thousandth of a gram (1,000 mg = 1 gm.)*
- *Microgram (mcg)—a unit of weight that equals one thousandth of a milligram or one millionth of a gram (1,000,000 mcg = 1 gm.)*

What's an International Unit (I.U.)? It's a standardized unit of measure based on the biological effect of a substance. Each I.U. of a vitamin has the same potency and action as another unit of the same vitamin.

Other minerals

Your body uses a large number of minerals. The trick is isolating them and determining what role, if any, they play in keeping you healthy. A couple of minerals —*chlorine* and *sulfur*—come in fairly high quantities in your body (both are bulk minerals) and yet are still mysterious (don't worry about getting enough: you get chlorine with any salt you eat, and sulfur is mixed in with most proteins). Trace minerals such as *tin*, *vanadium* (both touted for their importance in growth and development), and *molybdenum* have been isolated and considered potentially vital, yet for what no one is exactly sure. In the future we may even find out what roles minerals such as nickel, cadmium, gold, and lead play in the workings of the human machine.

Who's exposed to too much zinc?

Zinc plays a vital role in many normal body functions. So obviously, a zinc deficiency can impair the body's metabolism, growth, and development. But overexposure to zinc can also cause serious problems. Although zinc overexposure, or toxicity, is rare (except in people who overdose on supplements), it may appear in people who inhale zinc oxide dust or fumes in the following industries and occupations:

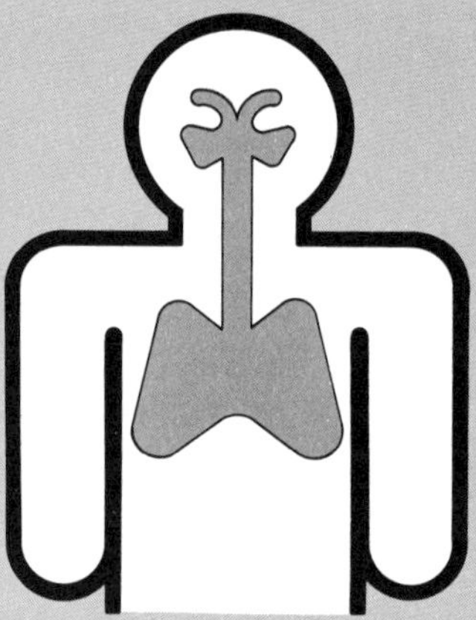

- *Alloy manufacturing*
- *Brass foundry work*
- *Bronze foundry work*
- *Electric fuse manufacturing*
- *Gas welding*
- *Electroplating*
- *Galvanizing*
- *Junk metal refining*
- *Paint manufacturing*
- *Metal cutting*
- *Metal spraying*
- *Rubber manufacturing*
- *Roof making*
- *Zinc manufacturing*

2 Getting your vitamins and minerals

Getting your recommended daily allowances
Once you know your recommended daily allowances (RDAs) for vitamins and minerals, you need to decide how to get them. Here are your options:
- *You can get your RDAs entirely from your diet, if you eat well-balanced meals of carefully chosen and prepared foods. This option is more natural and less expensive than the other option. It also provides other nutrients not listed on the RDA charts.*
- *You can add vitamin and mineral supplements to your diet. Although this method is more costly and less organic, it guarantees getting the RDAs even if your diet isn't ideal.*

You've seen it on the side of a box of cereal or even on a bag of potato chips—a list of how many calories and how much protein, fat, carbohydrates, cholesterol, and sodium are in any given serving. There's also a list of vitamins and minerals, showing what percentage of your daily dietary nutritional needs of each nutrient a serving provides. This second list is headed "US RDA"; RDA stands for Recommended Daily Allowances.

What you need

The RDAs for vitamins and minerals were established by the Food and Nutrition Board of the National Research Council. The board defines the RDAs as "the level of intake of essential nutrients considered, in the judgment of the Committee on Dietary Allowances of the Food and Nutrition Board on the basis of available scientific knowledge, to be adequate to meet the known nutritional needs of practically all healthy persons." This statement means that the RDAs are the *average* daily amounts—*not the minimum daily requirements*—for healthy people. The RDAs don't consider the special needs of people with metabolic disorders, chronic diseases, or infections, or of those who must take medications that may increase their nutritional needs. But many nutritionists, noting that the levels were set for *healthy* people, argue that the levels are too low for most of us and that for any of a dozen different reasons, people generally require more than the RDAs. Their feeling is that, while the RDAs are fine for many people, they're not necessarily what you need. You might need more potassium if you're an athlete, more Vitamin C if you smoke, more iron and calcium if you're a woman over 30, and so on. Or, quite possibly, you might need less than the RDAs. As one nutrition expert put it, saying the RDAs are all anyone needs is like saying all people should get "x" amount of oxygen each day, when in fact each person may need more or less oxygen than the next person.

When you look at the RDA chart, you'll notice that some RDAs differ according to a person's age and sex. Infants, children, and women generally require slightly less than male adults, while teenagers and pregnant women generally require slightly more. (Special needs of these groups are covered in later chapters of this book.)

Vitamin K and the more nebulous vitamins and minerals don't have established RDAs, either because the need for the vitamin or mineral is questioned, or, as in the case of Vitamin K, because a deficiency in the substance is highly unlikely.

Nevertheless, the RDAs provide useful information for working out your daily vitamin and mineral needs. In later chapters we'll discuss what your special needs may be.

As for the other vitamins and exotic trace minerals that you may hear about (such as vanadium and cadmium), don't worry about whether or not you're getting enough until scientists figure out what they actually do.

Don't let the numbers fool you

If you look through the tables the government publishes on the nutritive content of food, you'll find some interesting surprises: low on Vitamin A? A cup of heavy whipping cream will give you 3,500 I.U. (the RDA is 5,000 I.U.), a stick of butter 3,470 I.U., and a half-pound container of margarine 7,500 I.U. Want some more iron? How about eating an entire pecan pie—it'll give you 25.6 mg. of iron (the RDA is 18 mg.) In fact, the real "superfoods" according to the numbers are:

- Ice cream *(rich, hard), one-half gallon: 1,213 mg. calcium (RDA is 1,000 mg.), 927 mg phosphorus (RDA is 1,000 mg.), 7,200 I.U. Vitamin A (RDA is 5,000 I.U), 2.27 mg. riboflavin (RDA is 1.7 mg.).*
- Bread *(firm crumb), a two-pound loaf: 871 mg. calcium, 925 mg. phosphorus, 22.7 mg. iron, 3.60 mg. thiamine (RDA is 1.5 mg.), 2.20 mg. riboflavin, 30 mg. niacin (RDA is 20 mg.).*
- Cake, white *(two layers, with chocolate icing), eight or nine inches in diameter: 1,129 mg. calcium, 2,041 mg. phosphorus, 1.5 mg. thiamine, 1.77 mg. riboflavin, 12.5 mg. niacin.*

Of course, it's not likely you're going to sit down and polish off a two-pound loaf of bread. And if you ate the ice cream to get your daily dietary needs you'd end up the size of a house. This is why, when you check out the nutritive value of food, you should make sure the serving size used is reasonable. In other words—don't let the numbers fool you.

U.S. Recommended Daily Allowances (U.S. RDAs)

If you're in good health, use this chart to find out exactly what your needs are for the essential nutrients. If you have a health problem, ask your doctor how it affects your nutritional needs.

Nutrient and unit of measure‡	***Adults & children age 4 or older***	***Children under age 4***	***Infants under age 1***	***Pregnant or breast-feeding women***
*Vitamin A International Unit (I.U.)	5,000	2,500	1,500	8,000
Vitamin D International Unit (I.U.)	0400**	0400	0400	400
Vitamin E International Unit (I.U.)	30	10	5	30
*Vitamin C Milligrams (mg.)	60	40	35	60
Folic Acid Milligrams (mg.)	0.4	0.2	0.1	0.8
*Thiamine Milligrams (mg.)	1.5	0.7	0.5	1.7
*Riboflavin Milligrams (mg.)	1.7	0.8	0.6	2.0
*Niacin Milligrams (mg.)	20	9.0	8.0	20
Vitamin B_6 Milligrams (mg.)	2.0	0.7	0.4	2.5
Vitamin B_{12} Micrograms (mcg.)	6.0	3.0	2.0	8.0
Biotin Milligrams (mg.)	0.3	0.15	0.5	0.3
Pantothenic Acid Milligrams (mg.)	10	5.0	3.0	10
*Calcium Grams (gm.)	1.0	0.8	0.6	1.3
Phosphorus Grams (gm.)	1.0	0.8	0.5	1.3
Iodine Micrograms (mcg.)	150	70	45	150
*Iron Milligrams (mg.)	18	10	15	18
Magnesium Milligrams (mg.)	400	200	70	450
Copper Milligrams (mg.)	2.0	1.0	0.6	2.0
Zinc Milligrams (mg.)	15	8.0	5.0	15
+Protein Grams (gm.)	45	20	18	65-75

**Manufacturer must list these nutrients on nutrition labels.*
***Vitamin D is optional in supplements for adults and children age 4 or older.*
+If protein quality is equal to or greater than high-quality milk protein.
‡For more information about these units of measure, see How vitamins measure up, page 21.

Standards of identity

You won't always see a list of ingredients on every product label you check. That's because the Food and Drug Administration has established "standards of identity" for certain foods. These standards are based on what the FDA says that consumers expect a particular food to be like. To meet the standard, a product must have all the ingredients the government requires. If that's all the product contains, its label doesn't need to spell out the ingredients. But if the product also has artificial flavorings, artificial colorings, or chemical preservatives, the label must say so.

To meet the demands of nutrition-savvy consumers, many manufacturers list product ingredients for foods covered by standards. These include:

Cacao products
Bakery products
Milk and cream
Cheeses and related products
Frozen desserts
Nonartificial food flavorings
Dressings for foods
Canned and frozen fruits and fruit juices
Fruit butters, fruit jellies, fruit preserves, and related products
Shellfish and fish
Eggs and egg products
Oleomargarine, margarine
Nut products
Canned and frozen vegetables
Tomato products

Comparing labels

How can you tell a nutrition bargain from a nutrition bust? By comparing labels. Food labels aren't perfect, but, if you know how to read them, they'll tell you a lot about what a product contains. And by comparing labels of similar foods, you can choose the product that best suits your needs. For example, if you're trying to cut down on salt, you'll want to compare how much sodium different products have.

Also pay attention to the serving size listed on each label you compare. If you're watching your weight, a label that boasts "45 calories a serving" may sound great compared to one that lists 180 calories

NUTRITION INFORMATION
(PER SERVING)
SERVING SIZE = 1/2 CUP
SERVINGS PER CONTAINER = 1

CALORIES	280
PROTEIN	11 G
CARBOHYDRATE	21 G
FAT (PERCENT OF CALORIES 53%)	16 G
POLYUNSATURATED	1 G
SATURATED	4 G
CHOLESTEROL* (20 MG/100 G)	20 MG
SODIUM (365 MG/100 G)	415 MG

PERCENTAGE OF U.S. RECOMMENDED DAILY ALLOWANCES (U.S. RDAs)

PROTEIN	17
VITAMIN A	17
VITAMIN C (ASCORBIC ACID)	5
THIAMINE (VITAMIN B_1)	7
RIBOFLAVIN	7
NIACIN	12
CALCIUM	1
IRON	12

*Information on fat and cholesterol contents is provided for individuals who, on the advice of a physician, are modifying their total dietary intake of fat and cholesterol.

A label may include optional listings for cholesterol, fatty acids, and sodium.

How to read nutritional labels

First, it depends on what you're looking for. If you're looking at a bag of nacho chips, don't expect to find your RDA of vitamins and minerals. With junk food like that, your big concern will be calories, protein, carbohydrates, fats, cholesterol and salt. For that information you look to the top half of the label. If you're interested in what the product's made of, check the ingredients list. The government requires food manufacturers to state all ingredients a product contains, unless that product has been assigned a "standard of identity"—a definition of the food, based on certain standardized ingredients. Labels list ingredients in order of their weight, from the highest to lowest, with the main ingredients heading the list. When you want to find out what vitamins and minerals the food has, look to the lower half of the label. You'll find vitamins and minerals the government says must be listed on every package. Again, the ones that have to be there are vitamins A, C, B_1 (thiamine), B_2 (riboflavin), B_3 (niacin), calcium, and iron. Among others often listed are vitamins D, E, B_6, B_{12}, and phosphorus, magnesium, copper, and zinc. What you're looking for on the label is the column that states the percentages of the RDA for each nutrient in each serving.

a serving—until you realize that the serving size listed on the second label is four times as large as the one listed on the first label. (That means you'd eat 180 calories in equal servings of either product.)

Some labels offer more complete nutritional information than others. For example, one label may specify that a product contains "pepper, basil, and oregano"—ingredients that another label may simply group together as "natural flavorings." If you're allergic to certain flavors, colors, or spices, you'll want to look for labels with a detailed breakdown of individual ingredients.

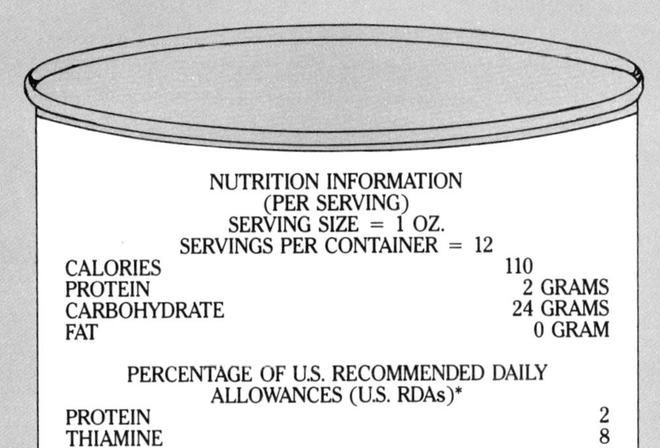

This is the minimum information that must appear on a nutrition label.

Servings in the four food groups

How much food is in a serving exactly? It all depends. In the milk group, the standard serving is an 8-ounce cup of whole milk. Alternate foods in the milk group are based on this standard.

They include:

1 cup nonfat milk
1 cup buttermilk
½ cup undiluted evaporated milk
¼ cup dried nonfat milk powder
¼ cup dried whole milk powder
1⅓ oz. cheddar, American, or Swiss cheese
16 oz. cream cheese
1⅓ cups cottage cheese
1⅔ cups ice cream
3 cups milk sherbet

So if you eat a cup of sherbet, count it as a third of a milk serving.

In the meat group, a serving can be 2 to 3 ounces of cooked meat, fish, or poultry. Or it can be 2 eggs, 1 cup of cooked dry beans, peas, or lentils, or 4 tablespoons of peanut butter.

For fruits and vegetables, the standard serving is ½ cup or 1 average portion, such as 1 medium apple or half of a grapefruit.

A serving in the bread-cereal group varies. It's a slice of bread, 1 ounce of ready-to-eat cereal, or ½ to ¾ cup of cooked cereal, cornmeal, grits, macaroni noodles, rice, or spaghetti.

How to meet your needs

The best way to meet your daily dietary needs of vitamins and minerals is through the food you eat. Ever since we were children we've been told we should have a balanced diet. Just what does that mean?

Every day a certain amount of your food should come from each of the four basic food groups:

• *Milk group.* This group not only includes milk in all of its forms (whole, skim, evaporated, dry, and buttermilk), but also encompasses cheese (cottage, cream, and natural or processed hard cheese) and ice cream. The recommended servings are listed in numbers of 8-ounce cups of whole milk daily:

Children under age 9	2 to 3 cups
Children age 9 to 12	3 or more cups
Teenagers	4 or more cups
Adults	2 or more cups
Pregnant women	3 or more cups
Nursing mothers	4 or more cups

• *Meat group.* In this food group, you'll find red meats, such as beef, veal, pork, and lamb, as well as poultry, fish, and eggs. Alternate choices in the meat group are dried beans, dried peas, and nuts. To help balance your diet, you need 2 or more servings from this group daily.

• *Fruit-vegetable group.* All types of fruits and vegetables belong to this basic food group. Although you need four or more servings every day, you should choose them carefully. Select at least one serving each day that's a good source of Vitamin C, and one serving at least every other day that's a good source of Vitamin A.

• *Bread-cereal group.* Your daily intake from the bread-cereal group should include four or more servings of whole grain, enriched, or restored breads; grain-derived products like pasta; and cereals, including oats, rice, millet, and barley, for example.

Building meals around the four food groups doesn't mean that you can't eat anything else. In fact, you'll probably want to add some fats, oils, sugars, refined flour, and spices to round out meals and to satisfy your appetite and calorie needs.

The recommendations put out by the National Research Council speak in terms of "servings." A rough, average serving size for a 1,200-calorie-a-day diet is four ounces, whether it be milk, cheese, meat, fruit, or cereal. If you have two four-ounce servings of meat a day, you should also have four ounces from the milk group and eight ounces each from the fruit-vegetable and grain groups. Many Americans eat a good deal more than that a day, so servings will be proportionately larger, depending on what you need.

The vitamins and minerals in food

Here's a look at each of the vitamins and minerals you need, showing you what foods they can be found in and how much those foods contain. Remember, just because a food is high in certain vitamins doesn't mean you should eat it all the time. There are other things to take into consideration when planning a menu. Even though liver is a "superfood," with a variety of vitamins and minerals, it's also rather high in calories and cholesterol, so you should substitute for liver occasionally—or skip it entirely if you can't stand the taste of it.

You can build a balanced diet by basing it on the four food groups. Within that rather broad structure you'll have a great deal of choice, and your choice should be guided by your desire to meet as much of your nutritional needs as possible through the foods you eat.

How to measure a serving

Most people estimate the size of a serving. But if you're watching your weight closely or if you just can't picture the size of a 4-ounce cooked hamburger, you may want to follow these tips:

- *Invest in a small scale to weigh your portions. Weigh your hamburger or other meat before and after you cook it. You'll see that it shrinks in size and weight after cooking. You can also use your scale to weigh out the correct serving of cereals, grains, and other foods.*
- *Look at the size of produce carefully when you shop and try to get an idea of medium or average sizes. For instance, an apple can be extra large—the kind that you see in a "bon voyage" fruit basket—or it can be small—almost the size of a plum.*
- *Measure foods with a measuring cup and measuring spoons. For accuracy, don't use a "heaping" teaspoon or cup. Instead, level it off. If you're using a see-through measuring cup, hold it at eye level to measure more precisely.*
- *Practice estimating the size of a serving. Be sure to confirm your guesses by weighing or measuring the food. You should soon be able to estimate a serving size with accuracy.*

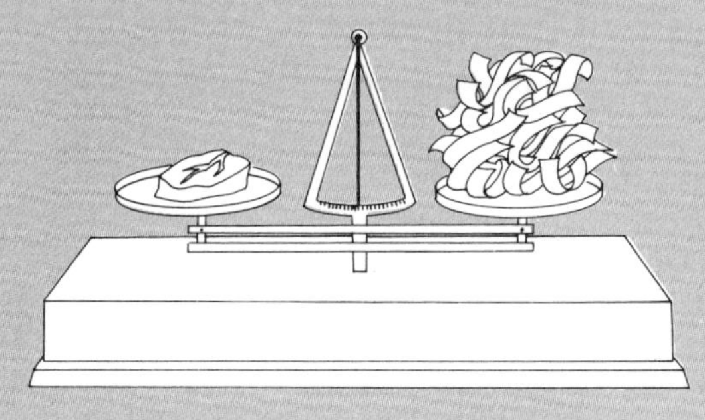

4 ounces of meat and 4 ounces of shredded carrots

Vitamins and minerals: their functions and food sources

Nutrient	Nutrient partners	Important functions
Vitamin A 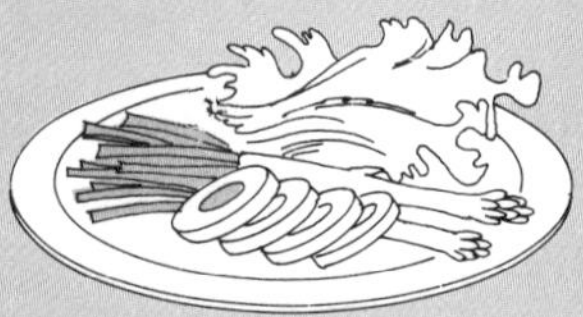 Good sources of Vitamin A include leaf lettuce, asparagus, and hard-boiled eggs.	B complex, Vitamin C, Vitamin D, Vitamin E, calcium, phosphorus, and zinc	Necessary for good vision, especially at night, healthy mucous membranes, skin, tooth development, and adrenal gland function. Essential for normal growth in children.
Thiamine (B_1) 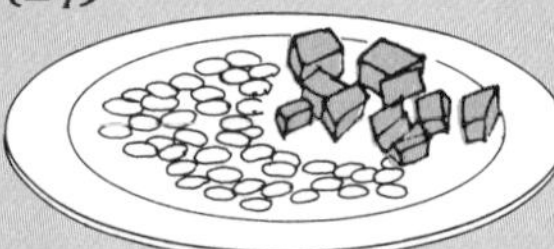 Vitamin B_1 needs daily replacement. Beef kidney and navy beans are good dietary sources of this vitamin.	B complex, Vitamin C, Vitamin E, and phosphorus	Necessary for growth, normal functioning of the brain, heart, nerves, and muscles, and for carbohydrate metabolism (chemical processes in the body that change food into energy and living tissue)
Riboflavin (B_2) Certain common foods can supply your daily requirement for Vitamin B_2. Those shown here are whole milk, Swiss cheese, and white meat of chicken.	B complex, Vitamin C, and phosphorus	Necessary for growth, normal eye and nervous system function, healthy skin and mucous membranes, and carbohydrate metabolism

Food source	*Portion*	*Nutrient amount*	*RDA**
Beef liver	*3 oz.*	*45,390 (I.U.)*	*5,000 International Units (I.U.)*
Sweet potato	*1 medium*	*11,904*	
Carrots	*½ cup*	*8,140*	
Spinach, cooked	*½ cup*	*7,290*	
Cantaloupe	*¼ medium*	*4,620*	
Broccoli, cooked	*1 stalk*	*4,500*	
Squash, winter	*½ cup*	*4,305*	
Apricots, fresh	*3 medium*	*2,890*	
Watermelon	*1 slice*	*2,510*	
Peach	*1 medium*	*1,300*	
Tomato	*1 medium*	*1,100*	
Leaf lettuce	*1 cup*	*1,050*	
Asparagus, cooked	*4 spears*	*540*	
Peas, cooked	*½ cup*	*430*	
Green beans	*½ cup*	*340*	
Egg, hard-boiled	*1 large*	*260*	
Sunflower seeds	*¼ cup*	*0.7 (mg)*	*1.5 mg*
Soybeans	*¼ cup*	*0.6*	
Wheat germ	*1 oz.*	*0.6*	
Beef kidney	*3 oz.*	*0.4*	
Ham, baked	*3 oz.*	*0.4*	
Navy beans	*¼ cup*	*0.3*	
Salmon steak	*3 oz.*	*0.2*	
Rice, brown	*¼ cup*	*0.2*	
Beef liver	*3 oz.*	*0.2*	
Yogurt, lowfat plain	*8 oz.*	*0.1*	
Beef kidney	*3 oz.*	*4.1 (mg)*	*1.7 mg*
Beef liver	*3 oz.*	*3.6*	
Chicken liver	*3 oz.*	*1.5*	
Milk, whole	*1 cup*	*0.4*	
Milk, skim	*1 cup*	*0.4*	
Lamb, roasted	*3 oz.*	*0.3*	
Chicken, white meat	*3 oz.*	*0.3*	
Swiss cheese	*2 oz.*	*0.2*	
Beef, lean	*3 oz.*	*0.2*	

**U.S. Recommended Daily Allowances for adults and children age 4 and over.*

Continued

Vitamins and minerals: their functions and food sources

(continued)

Nutrient	Nutrient partners	Important functions
Niacin (B_3) 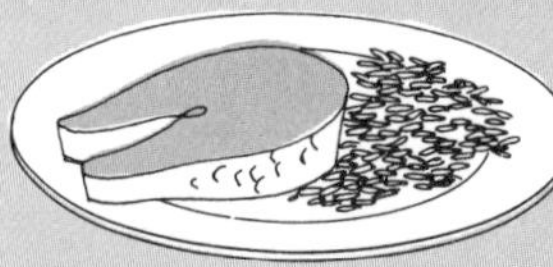 *Salmon and peanuts are two examples of Vitamin B_3-rich foods.*	*B complex, Vitamin C, and phosphorus*	*Necessary for healthy skin and normal functioning of the stomach and intestines, the nervous system, and the circulatory system. Vitamin B_3 also aids carbohydrate, fat, and protein metabolism.*
Vitamin B_6 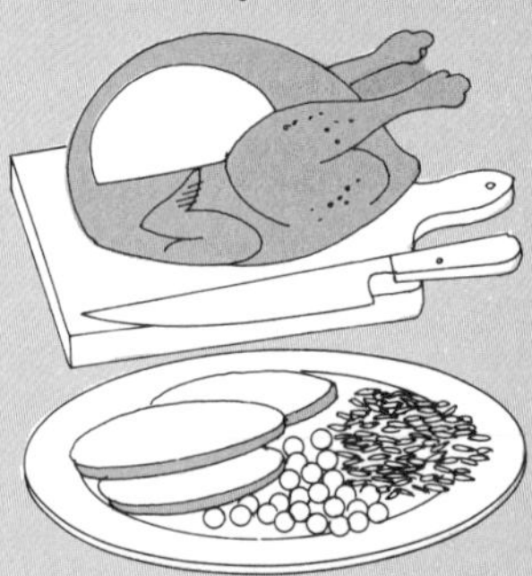 *Major sources of Vitamin B_6 are white chicken meat, chick peas, and sunflower seeds.*	*B complex, pantothenic acid, Vitamin C, magnesium, potassium, and sodium*	*Necessary for fat, carbohydrate, and protein metabolism. Essential for growth and replacement of red blood cells. Maintains normal functioning of nervous system.*
Vitamin B_{12} 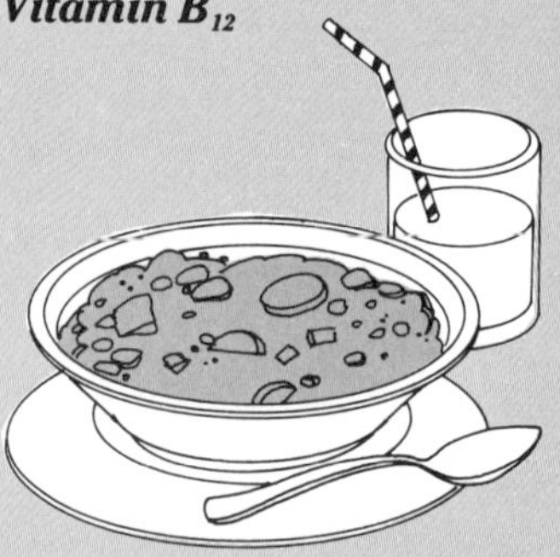 *Vitamin B_{12} is found in animal products only. Beef kidney stew and whole milk are two good examples.*	*B complex, folic acid, Vitamin C, potassium, and sodium*	*Necessary for healthy nervous system and iron metabolism. Also aids circulation.*

Food source	Portion	Nutrient amount	RDA*
Beef liver	3 oz.	14.0 (mg)	20 mg
Tuna, canned, in oil	½ cup	12.0	
Chicken, white meat	3 oz.	10.6	
Beef kidney	3 oz.	9.1	
Salmon steak	3 oz.	8.4	
Peanuts, chopped	¼ cup	6.2	
Veal cutlet	3 oz.	4.5	
Beef, lean	3 oz.	3.9	
Chicken liver	3 oz.	3.8	
Rice, brown	¼ cup	2.4	
Salmon steak	3 oz.	0.6 (mg)	2.0 mg
Chicken, white meat	3 oz.	0.5	
Beef liver	3 oz.	0.5	
Chicken liver	3 oz.	0.5	
Sunflower seeds	¼ cup	0.5	
Soybeans	¼ cup	0.4	
Chick peas	¼ cup	0.3	
Rice, brown	¼ cup	0.3	
Beef liver	3 oz.	49.6 (mcg)	6.0 micrograms (mcg)
Clams, canned	½ cup	20.0	
Beef kidney	3 oz.	19.0	
Chicken liver	3 oz.	16.5	
Salmon, canned	½ cup	7.6	
Salmon steak	3 oz.	3.0	
Beef, lean	3 oz.	1.4	
Swiss cheese	2 oz.	1.0	
Milk, whole	1 cup	0.9	
Egg, hard-boiled	1	0.7	
Chicken, white meat	3 oz.	0.3	

*U.S. Recommended Daily Allowances for adults and children age 4 and over.

Continued

Vitamins and minerals: their functions and food sources

(continued)

Nutrient	Nutrient partners	Important functions
Folic acid 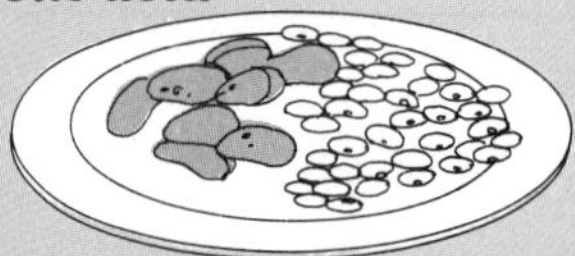 *Three ounces of chicken livers supply more than the U.S. RDA for folic acid. Kidney beans are another source of this vitamin.*	*B complex and Vitamin C*	*Necessary for protein metabolism and tissue growth and development. Folic acid also helps produce red blood cells and helps convert some amino acids to other kinds of amino acids.*
Vitamin C 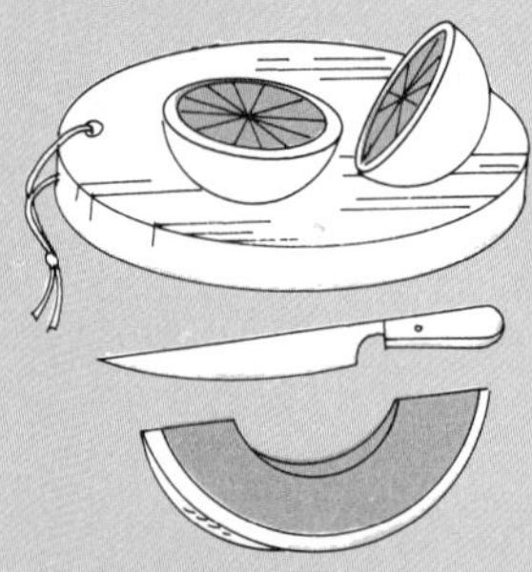 *Because your body can't store it, Vitamin C must be consumed daily in such foods as oranges and cantaloupes.*	*All vitamins and minerals, especially calcium and magnesium*	*Necessary for growth, tooth and gum development, iron absorption, protein metabolism, and healing of wounds and burns, Vitamin C also keeps blood vessels strong. Keeps blood free of clots.*
Vitamin D 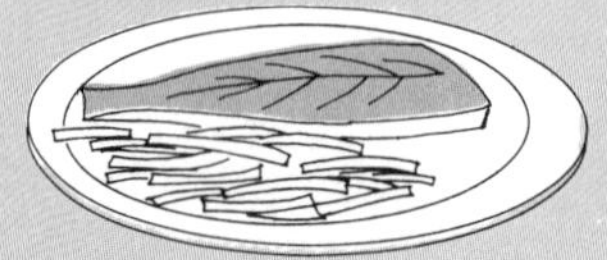 *Oil from several types of fish is a good source of Vitamin D.*	*Vitamin A, Vitamin C, calcium, and phosphorus*	*Helps in absorption and use of calcium and phosphorus. Vitamin D is essential for good bone structure and tooth development.*

Food source	Portion	Nutrient amount	RDA*
Chicken liver	3 oz.	0.65 (mg)	0.4 mg
Beef liver	3 oz.	0.12	
Chick peas	¼ cup	0.10	
Soybeans	¼ cup	0.09	
Sunflower seeds	¼ cup	0.08	
Navy beans	¼ cup	0.07	
Kidney beans	¼ cup	0.06	
Beef kidney	3 oz.	0.05	
Peanuts, chopped	¼ cup	0.04	
Orange juice, fresh squeezed	1 cup	124 (mg)	60 mg
Green peppers, raw, chopped	½ cup	96	
Grapefruit juice, fresh squeezed	1 cup	94	
Brussels sprouts	4 sprouts	73	
Broccoli, raw, chopped	½ cup	70	
Orange	1 medium	70	
Cantaloupe	¼ medium	56	
Cauliflower, raw, chopped	½ cup	45	
Strawberries	½ cup	42	
Grapefruit	½ medium	41	
Honeydew	⅛	40	
Tomato juice	1 cup	39	
Potato, baked	1 medium	31	
Tomato	1 medium	28	
Pineapple	1 cup	25	
Cabbage, raw, chopped	½ cup	21	
Blackberries	½ cup	15	
Spinach, raw, chopped	½ cup	14	
Lettuce, romaine	1 cup	10	
Halibut-liver oil	2 tsp.	11,200 (I.U.)	400 I.U.
Herring	3 oz.	840	
Cod-liver oil	2 tsp.	800	
Mackerel	3 oz.	708	
Salmon, Pacific	3 oz.	420	
Tuna	2 oz.	168	

*U.S. Recommended Daily Allowances for adults and children age 4 and over.

Continued

Vitamins and minerals: their functions and food sources

(continued)

Nutrient	*Nutrient partners*	*Important functions*
Vitamin E 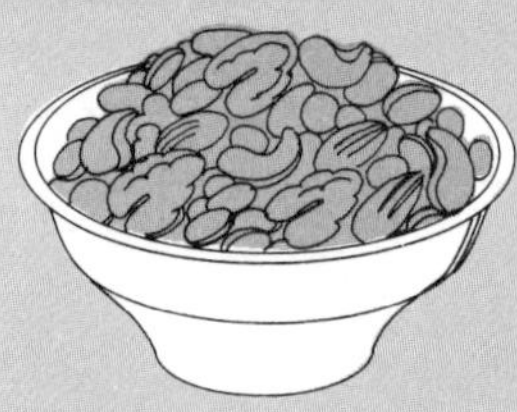 *Most foods contain Vitamin E. Nuts are a good source.*	*Vitamin A, B complex, Vitamin C, manganese, selenium, and phosphorus*	*Protects red blood cells from damage and degeneration. Prevents blood clotting within veins. Stops abnormal breakdown of fatty acids.*
Calcium 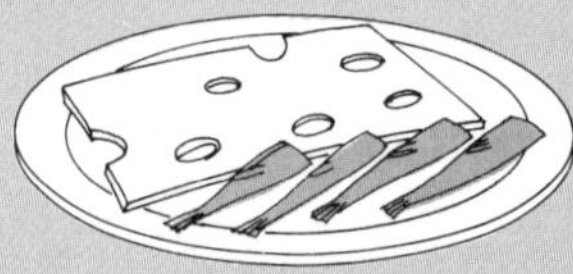 *At every stage of life, your body needs calcium-rich foods, such as cheese and other dairy products.*	*Vitamin A, Vitamin C, Vitamin D, iron, magnesium, manganese, and phosphorus*	*Essential for bone and tooth formation, blood clotting, cardiovascular health, and normal muscle and nervous system activity*
Iron 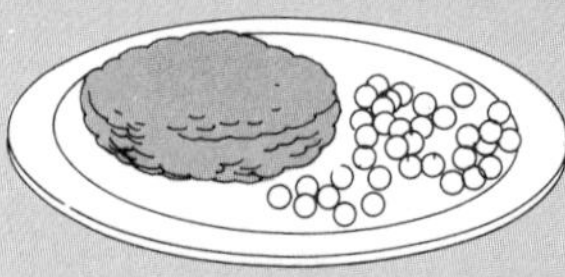 *A small serving of ground beef and peas can supply a significant amount of your body's iron requirement.*	*Vitamin B_{12}, folic acid, Vitamin C, calcium, and phosphorus*	*Combines with protein to form hemoglobin, which carries oxygen to the tissues*

Food source	Portion	Nutrient amount	RDA*
Wheat germ oil	1 tbsp.	37.2 (I.U.)	30 I.U.
Sunflower seeds	¼ cup	26.8	
Wheat germ, raw	½ cup	12.8	
Sunflower seed oil	1 tbsp.	12.7	
Almonds	¼ cup	12.7	
Pecans	¼ cup	12.5	
Hazelnuts	¼ cup	12.0	
Safflower oil	1 tbsp.	7.9	
Peanuts	¼ cup	4.9	
Corn oil	1 tbsp.	4.8	
Cod-liver oil	1 tbsp.	3.9	
Peanut butter	2 tbsp.	3.8	
Corn oil margine	1 tbsp.	3.6	
Soybean oil	1 tbsp.	3.5	
Peanut oil	1 tbsp.	3.4	
Swiss cheese	2 oz.	544 (mg)	1.0 gram
Yogurt, skim milk	1 cup	452	
Monterey Jack cheese	2 oz.	424	
Cheddar cheese	2 oz.	408	
Colby cheese	2 oz.	388	
Brick cheese	2 oz.	382	
Sardines, Atlantic, drained	3 oz.	371	
Mozzarella cheese	2 oz.	366	18 mg
American cheese	2 oz.	348	
Milk, skim	1 cup	302	
Milk, whole	1 cup	288	
Buttermilk	1 cup	285	
Salmon, sockeye, drained	3 oz.	274	
Broccoli, cooked	1 medium stalk	158	
Cheese spread	1 oz.	158	
Pizza, cheese	1 slice	144	
Blackstrap molasses	1 tbsp.	137	
Ice milk	½ cup	120	
Ice cream	½ cup	110	
Beef liver	3 oz.	7.5 (mg)	
Beef kidney	2 oz.	4.7	
Clams	2 oz.	4.2	
Oysters, raw	2 oz.	3.4	

*U.S. Recommended Daily Allowances for adults and children age 4 and over.

Continued

Vitamins and minerals: their functions and food sources
(continued)

Nutrient	*Nutrient partners*	*Important functions*
Iron *(cont.)*		
Potassium 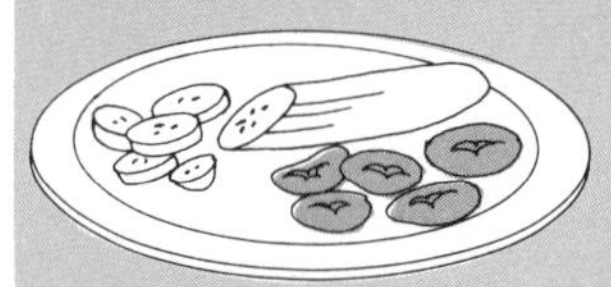 *The usual intake of potassium is 2,000 to 4,000 mg per day. Bananas, dried apricots, and prunes are all good dietary sources of this nutrient.*	*Vitamin B_6 and sodium*	*Aids muscle contraction, nerve transmission, water and chemical balance in the body, and enzyme action*

Food source	Portion	Nutrient amount	RDA*
Blackstrap molasses	1 tbsp.	3.2	18 mg
Roast beef	3 oz.	3.1	
Ground beef	3 oz.	3.0	
Lima beans, dried, cooked	½ cup	2.9	
Sunflower seeds	¼ cup	2.6	
Veal, roasted	2 oz.	2.2	
Turkey, dark meat	3 oz.	2.0	
Apricots, dried	¼ cup	1.8	
Broccoli, raw	1 stalk	1.7	
Spinach, raw, chopped	1 cup	1.7	
Almonds, slivered	¼ cup	1.6	
Peas, fresh, cooked	½ cup	1.5	
Raisins	¼ cup	1.3	
Chicken, white meat	3 oz.	1.0	
Potato	1 medium	782 (mg)	RDA not established
Avocado	½ medium	602	
Raisins	½ cup	545	
Sardines, Atlantic, drained	3 oz.	501	
Flounder	3 oz.	498	
Orange juice	1 cup	496	
Squash, winter	½ cup	473	
Banana	1 medium	451	
Apricots, dried	¼ cup	448	
Tomato, raw	1 medium	444	
Milk, skim	1 cup	406	
Cantaloupe	½	400	
Salmon, fillet, fresh, cooked	3 oz.	378	
Milk, whole	1 cup	370	
Prunes, dried, raw	5	355	
Beef liver	3 oz.	323	
Peach	1 medium	308	
Grapefruit juice, canned	¾ cup	300	
Round steak, trimmed of fat	3 oz.	298	
Pork, trimmed of fat	3 oz.	283	
Lamb, trimmed of fat	3 oz.	274	
Celery, raw	2 large stalks	270	
Orange	1 medium	270	
Turkey, white meat	3 oz.	259	
Turkey, dark meat	3 oz.	247	
Tuna, drained solids	3 oz.	225	

*U.S. Recommended Daily Allowances for adults and children age 4 and over.

Continued

Vitamins and minerals: their functions and food sources
(continued)

Nutrient	Nutrient partners	Important functions
Magnesium 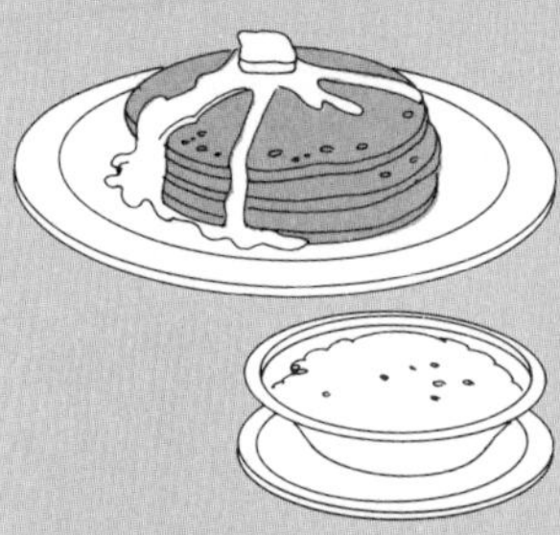 *Whole grain products, such as oatmeal and pancakes made from buckwheat flour, are high in magnesium*	*Vitamin B_6, Vitamin C, Vitamin D, calcium, and phosphorus*	*Activates many enzymes. Regulates cell metabolism and growth. Magnesium also aids muscle and nerve function.*
Zinc 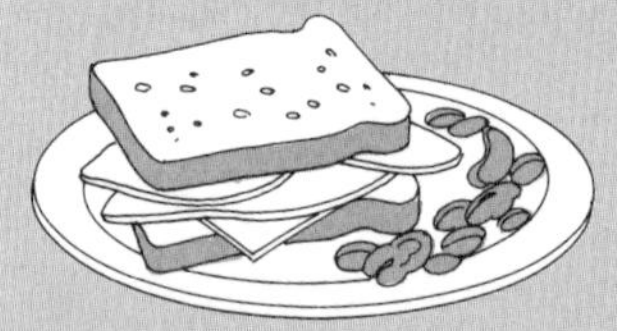 *Lean beef and nuts are good sources of zinc.*	*Vitamin A, calcium, and phosphorus*	*A component of insulin and of many enzyme systems involved in activities such as growth, reproduction, and wound healing.*

Food source	*Portion*	*Nutrient amount*	*RDA**
Soy flour	*½ cup*	*155 (mg)*	*400 mg*
Soybeans, dried	*¼ cup*	*138*	
Grapefruit	*½*	*128*	
Cucumber, raw, peeled	*½*	*125*	
Buckwheat flour, light	*½ cup*	*112*	
Almonds, whole	*¼ cup*	*96*	
Cashews	*¼ cup*	*95*	
Kidney beans, dried, cooked	*¼ cup*	*82*	
Lima beans, dried, raw	*¼ cup*	*81*	
Brazil nuts	*¼ cup*	*79*	
Pecans	*¼ cup*	*77*	
Whole wheat flour	*½ cup*	*68*	
Shredded wheat	*1 cup*	*67*	
Peanuts, roasted	*¼ cup*	*63*	
Walnuts, black	*¼ cup*	*60*	
Banana	*1 medium*	*58*	
Avocado	*½ medium*	*56*	
Peanut butter	*2 tbsp.*	*56*	
Blackstrap molasses	*1 tbsp.*	*52*	
Potato	*1 medium*	*51*	
Oatmeal	*1 cup*	*50*	
Chicken heart	*3 oz.*	*6.3 (mg)*	*15 mg*
Beef, lean	*3 oz.*	*5.3*	
Calves' liver	*3 oz.*	*5.2*	
Beef liver	*3 oz.*	*4.4*	
Lamb, lean	*3 oz.*	*4.3*	
Ground beef, lean	*3 oz.*	*3.8*	
Chicken liver	*3 oz.*	*3.7*	
Turkey, dark meat	*3 oz.*	*3.5*	
Pumpkin seeds	*¼ cup*	*2.6*	
Chicken, dark meat	*3 oz.*	*2.4*	
Swiss cheese	*2 oz.*	*2.2*	
Sunflower seeds	*¼ cup*	*2.0*	
Brazil nuts	*¼ cup*	*1.8*	
Cheddar cheese	*2 oz.*	*1.8*	
Turkey, white meat	*3 oz.*	*1.8*	

**U.S. Recommended Daily Allowances for adults and children age 4 and over.*

Other vitamins and the foods they're in

There are no specific figures available for these:

Biotin: Liver and other organ meats, egg yolk, peanuts, filberts, mushrooms, cauliflower, various fruits, unpolished rice.

Pantothenic acid: Organ meats, egg yolk, peanuts, broccoli, cauliflower, cabbage, whole grains.

Choline: Most B-complex sources.

Inositol: Most B-complex sources.

PABA: Other B-complex sources.

Other minerals and the foods they're in

There are no specific figures available for these:

Chromium: Calves' liver, potatoes (with skin), whole grains, beef, cheese, fresh vegetables, chicken legs, fresh fruit, seafood, chicken breasts.

Copper: Nuts, organ meats, seafood, mushrooms, peas, legumes.

Fluoride (fluorine): Drinking water.

Iodine: Table salt.

Manganese: Whole grains, wheat germ, peas, tea, ginger, beets, egg yolk.

Phosphorus: Meat, fish, poultry, eggs, milk, cheese, nuts.

Selenium: Wheat germ, organ meats, tuna, onions, tomatoes, broccoli.

Silicon: Most natural foods, beer.

Sodium (salt): Bacon, tomatoes, cottage cheese, and most other foods.

How to keep vitamins and minerals in your food

Avoid processed foods as much as possible. Processing food so it can travel great distances and last a long time on a store's shelf takes a great toll on it, robbing it of many of its essential nutrients. Take B_6. There's a fair amount of it in whole-grain products, but once that grain has been turned into shredded wheat, 38 percent is gone. And that's not freezing it or canning it—just processing it. And the loss of vitamins gets worse. By the time that same grain becomes white bread, 78 percent of the B_6 has vanished, and when it gets refined

Preserving the nutrients

Some food preparation methods can strip foods of their nutrients. But you can preserve most of the vitamins and minerals, if you follow these guidelines:

- *Eat raw fruits and vegetables. When you must cut or trim them, do it as little as possible and just before you cook or eat them. Remember, a sliced cucumber loses a third of its vitamin C in an hour. One-inch pieces of cooked green beans lose much less vitamin C than French-cut beans sliced lengthwise.*
- *Rinse fresh produce just enough to remove dirt.*
- *Soak dried beans and peas until they're slightly softened.*
- *Never wash white rice. A single rinsing can rob you of a quarter of its thiamine.*
- *Avoid boiling vegetables for a long time in lots of water. Boiling can destroy up to 80% of the vitamin C and dissolve other water-soluble vitamins. Instead, try steaming your vegetables. This process can double the amount of nutrients that remain in broccoli and other vegetables. Or you may want to stir fry your vegetables—another nutrient-saving method. Whichever method you use, remember to cook vegetables until they're tender, in just enough liquid to prevent scorching.*
- *Use any excess cooking liquids as a base for soup or a sauce.*

to the point of cake flour, 87 percent has disappeared.

Processing isn't just a matter of mashing up and breaking down food. It can also involve adding preservatives, some of which render certain nutrients useless. If you must eat food that's been processed, go for what's frozen rather than what's canned, and be sure to read the nutritional information to see what you're getting.

Your best bet is to buy and prepare the freshest possible produce you can find. Get your meat from a local butcher, your vegetables and fruits from the neighborhood grocery store. Keep your eye out for things grown locally—the shorter the time between when a vegetable is picked and when you put it in your mouth, the better.

Even if you prepare all your own meals from the freshest food you can find, you can still destroy a number of vitamins by too much soaking or cooking. Eat some of your fruits and vegetables raw. Wash fruits and vegetables quickly.

With all this, you must think it's pretty well impossible to get your daily nutrient needs from even the most well-balanced diet. It's not unless your needs are higher than normal.

Special formulas for special needs

You can find a bewildering array of vitamin and mineral supplements in almost any drugstore, supermarket, or health food store. In addition to supplements for each individual vitamin and mineral, combinations exist to meet very specialized needs. So be sure to assess your needs before you try to select a supplement. Then look at the formulas before you decide to buy. Here are some common formulas that you're likely to find:

- *multivitamin*
- *multivitamin and multimineral*
- *multimineral*
- *multivitamin with iron*
- *Vitamin A and D*
- *Vitamin B complex*
- *Vitamin B complex and C*
- *stress vitamins.*

Are supplements necessary?

Do you *have* to take a vitamin pill to meet all your nutritional needs? The answer is no—you can probably get all you need from what you eat, but you have to eat sensibly. Still, beyond what you eat, you might have special needs.

If you're a woman, you're probably low in iron and calcium, but you might not want to eat lots of liver and cheese to get the iron and calcium for fear of also getting too much cholesterol or too many calories. If you smoke, you're going to need to make up for the Vitamin C that cigarettes take out of you. If you're a strict vegetarian, you're not getting much iron or any B_{12}. If you're taking prescription drugs, if you drink coffee, tea, or colas, if you're pregnant or a nursing mother, if you're over age 60, if...everyone has specific needs, so it's likely that somewhere along the line you'll fall into one or more groups of the vitamin and mineral needy.

If you think you should take a supplement, what should you take? Again, that all depends on you and your needs. In later sections we'll see that certain vitamins and minerals do certain things for you, and you might want to take specific supplements for specific purposes. To begin with, all you probably need is a basic multivitamin and multimineral supplement. Check the labels. The big national brands usually contain 100 percent of the RDAs for the essential vitamins and minerals. Drugstores and health food stores carry brands with two or three times the RDAs. Some experts say the extra is just a waste, while others feel those extra amounts do a great deal of good. One thing's for sure: you don't want insufficient intake of essential vitamins and minerals for any period of time.

How to choose a supplement
Before you choose a supplement, consider what you actually need or want. To pin down your needs, record the food that you eat every day for about a week. At the end of each day, estimate the nutrient value of the

Guide to supplements

If you decide to take vitamin and mineral supplements, and think you want something more than a big national brand, you're going to find yourself confronted by a baffling number of choices and alternatives. Here's a quick guide through the maze. Beware: *added features may just mean added cost, not added benefit.*

- Buffered: *Some Vitamin C products are buffered, which, as with aspirin, makes them easier on your stomach. You need buffered vitamins only if you have a very sensitive stomach.*

- Chelated *(pronounced key-lated): Chelated minerals are supposedly easier for your body to use. But they cost more, and if you take your supplement with your meals (as you should), your body will use the minerals just as well as if they were chelated.*

- Emulsified: *Only the fat-soluble vitamins, A, D, and E, come in emulsified forms. Fat-soluble vitamins are dissolved by fats in your body. Emulsification allows them to be dissolved by water. A good bet for people who don't digest oils and fats well.*

- Enzymes added: *Enzymes break down food. You already have them in your body, and unless you have very poor digestion, paying for extra enzymes is just paying for things you already own.*

- Timed release capsule, tablet, chewable, powdered: *Timed release seems like a great idea for those vitamins your body flushes out fairly quickly, like Vitamin C. But there's some indication the theory doesn't stand up in practice. Your body doesn't use as much of a timed-release dose as it does a tablet, chewable tablet, or powdered dose. In*

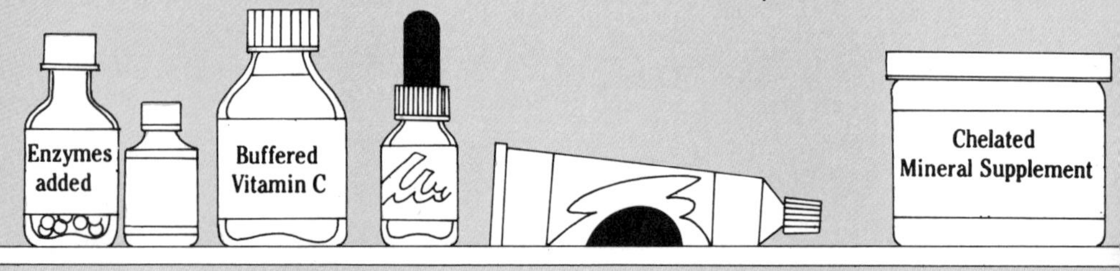

food, using the nutritional information of the package labels and in the chart on pages 30-41. Then add up your daily intake of vitamins and minerals, and compare it to the RDA.

If you're eating a well-balanced diet, you probably won't need a supplement. But if your diet lacks certain vitamins or minerals that you can't (or won't) get from eating nutrient-rich foods, you may want to consider a vitamin or mineral supplement.

When you shop for a supplement, consider your wants, too. Can you swallow one large pill, or do you need to take several smaller ones? Will you remember to take several pills every day? Do you want a supplement that you can chew? A supplement that's gentle to your stomach? The Guide to supplements can help you decide which forms are for you.

fact, it gets the most out of the powdered form, which also happens to be the cheapest. (When you can buy it—powdered vitamins are hard to find.)

- Organic: *This should mean something produced without the use of any chemicals, but there's no law regulating the use of the term, so there's a lot of stuff out there that says it's organic but really isn't. You'll find it hard to tell the real from the fake. "Organic" vitamins are probably not worth the extra cost.*
- Natural versus synthetic: The *debate in the vitamin world. Should you take vitamins made from a natural substance (like Vitamin C derived from rose hips) or vitamins created synthetically in a lab? Some say natural is the best route, while others point out that even natural vitamins are flooded with chemicals in the process of drawing them out of the original substance. Moreover, natural vitamins may contain as yet unanalyzed, perhaps beneficial, components; synthetics contain only what's put into them. Still, there's little evidence that naturals do the job any better, or, for that matter, that your body can tell the difference. Only your wallet can tell the difference—naturals cost a fair bit more than synthetics.*
- Types: *You'll notice that your vitamins and minerals may come in a variety of different types. For the most part this doesn't matter. Ascorbic acid is just as good as Vitamin C. However, in the case of iron and calcium there is a difference. In iron, you want ferrous, not ferric oxide (your body can't use ferric). In calcium, although bonemeal and dolomite are good sources, they may also have traces of lead, so go for either calcium gluconate or calcium carbonate.*

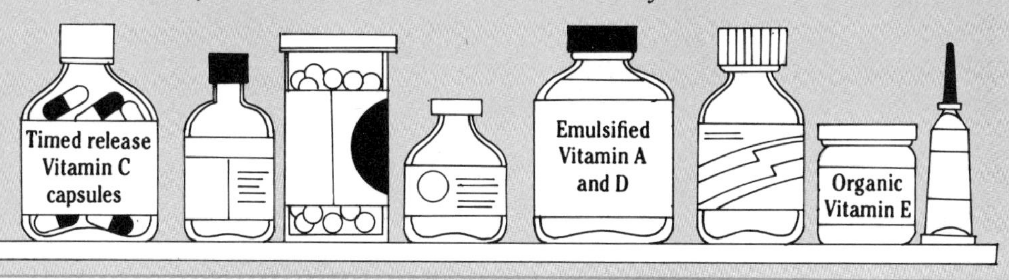

3 What vitamins and minerals can do

A look at night blindness
Because vitamin A is a vital part of the light-sensitive part of the eyes, a vitamin A deficiency can cause night blindness—vision difficulty in dim light.

The only diseases that vitamins and minerals can cure are those diseases—like scurvy—that are brought on by the complete absence of certain vitamins. But vitamins and minerals aren't noticed only by their absence—they're noticed by their presence, too. For example, the absence of Vitamin C can cause scurvy, but the presence of Vitamin C can do more than cure scurvy. When you get enough Vitamin C, it keeps your blood vessels strong and your tissues healthy, and it might even help ward off the common cold and other bugs.

Although they can't cure all the diseases that afflict us, vitamins and minerals can do a lot for us. In particular, they can help us feel healthy—and stay that way.

Here's a look at each of the major vitamins and minerals, showing what their presence in your diet can do for you.

Vitamin A

During World War II, the British, in an effort to keep the Germans uninformed about their newly developed radar technology, spread the rumor that British anti-aircraft gunners could see so well at night because they ate a lot of carrots. Although this story was a wartime hoax, the British were right—carrots do help you see better at night. They're high in Vitamin A, and A is a crucial component of the chemical in your eyes that lets you see at night and in dim light. But Vitamin A does more for you than just help you see better at night. It also keeps your skin healthy by stopping it from drying out, and it can help cuts and scrapes heal faster. Vitamin A also keeps your mucous membranes moist and functioning—and that's important: your mucous membranes are your body's first line of defense against incoming airborne bacteria, trapping particles before they can get into your lungs. Vitamin A, then, is on the front line of defense against everyday viruses and infections.

Vitamin A—the eyes have it

At the back of your eye is your retina. It's a field of sensors, rods and cones, each of which picks up a small part of the image that your lens focuses onto it. Your brain then takes all these tiny bits of image and fuses them together into one picture. But at the heart of how we see is how each rod and cone turns light into a message that the brain can understand. In each rod and cone is a chemical that, when struck by light, creates a small electrical charge that zips along your optic nerve to your brain. The chemical in the rods is a pigment known as rhodopsin, or visual purple, and one of its crucial components is Vitamin A.

As it happens, the cones are the sensors we use to see in bright light. They don't work in dim light, whereas that's the light the rods thrive on (in bright light they are blinded). If you become seriously deficient in Vitamin A, the rhodopsin can't do its job well and your ability to see in dim light and at night suffers. So watch your Vitamin A intake and see a doctor if you're having trouble with your eyes.

Parts of the eye

In the inner layer of your retina, the cones provide detailed color vision and work best in bright light. The rods provide vision in dim light. As darkness increases, vision shifts from cones to rods.

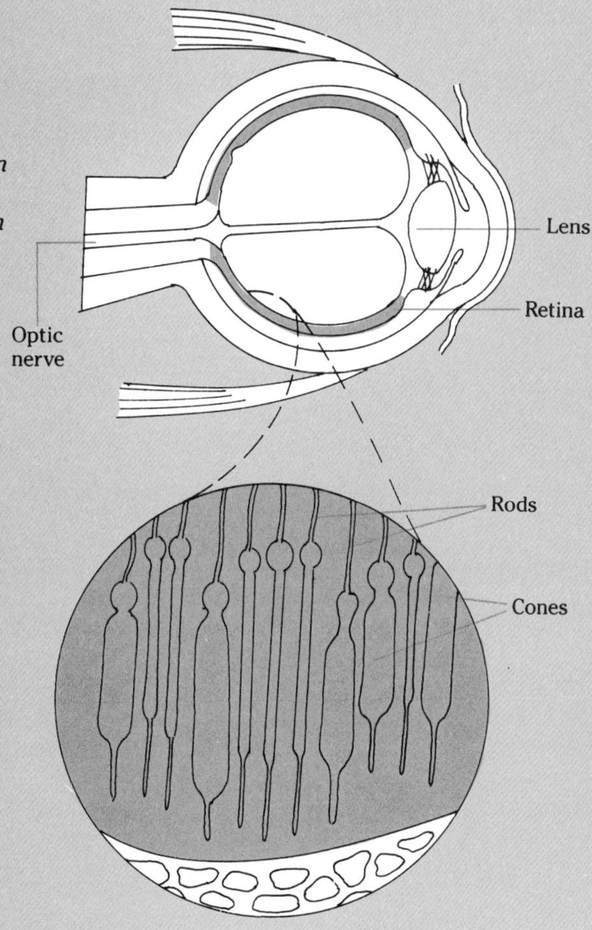

Chasing the blues away

Reed just hasn't been feeling his best lately. He thinks he's down because his career isn't going as well as he'd hoped. That may indeed be the reason. But it also may be that Reed has had precious little in the way of B-complex vitamins lately, and he hasn't been out in the sun for weeks.

Mental health doesn't just mean not *hearing voices; it also means feeling sharp and not being depressed. Some believe that even a slight deficiency in your B vitamins can leave you feeling a little less than your happiest. Some depression can be the direct result of serious deficiencies in iron and B_{12}. Some women taking contraceptive pills suffer from occasional bouts of depression, and many of them respond well to added B_6.*

Recent studies in Scandinavia report a connection between how much sunlight exposure we get (and how much Vitamin D we receive) and how happy we are. It seems that Vitamin D can defend you from depression.

B-complex vitamins

Originally, the B-complex vitamins were all thought to be one vitamin, and although they have all been found to be somewhat different chemically, they're all still related. They work synergistically—that is, they work better together as a team than they do on their own because what they do is interrelated. Still, each of the vitamins has its own specific role to play, and each can do something beneficial for you.

Thiamine

If your body were a car and carbohydrates were the gasoline, then thiamine would be the spark that ignites the fuel. In your body, the balance between your carbohydrate intake and the amount of thiamine present is precarious. Too little thiamine and you have carbohydrate overload. In that case, your body has a defense mechanism—it simply slows down, reducing your appetite so that you take in less fuel. Even this minor deficiency—a long way from the acute thiamine deficiency of beriberi—can lead to physical exhaustion. Getting all the thiamine you need will keep your engine running fine, giving you the energy you need. And this is all tied in with thiamine's role in ensuring smooth functioning of your brain and nervous system.

Riboflavin

Riboflavin plays another role in the process of igniting your body's fuel. Just as air is mixed with gas in a car's engine before it's ignited, so oxygen is mixed with carbohydrates. Riboflavin is part of the team that gets the oxygen to the carbohydrates. When your body's low in riboflavin, just as when it's low in thiamine, it can't get all the energy it needs. Fortunately, deficiency symptoms—including inflamed tongue, sore throat, cracked lips and corners of the mouth, dry patches of skin, eyes hypersensitive to light, nervousness, depression—can alert you to a deficiency. As with all the B vitamins, riboflavin can help keep you on a steady course, mentally and physically.

Niacin

The relationship between niacin deficiency and the mental illness brought on by pellagra has been established, and although there's some controversy here, many experts feel that even a small deficiency in this vitamin can affect our health, making us irritable and confused. A severe deficiency can affect the skin, nervous system, and digestive tract. As with thiamine and riboflavin, maintaining your RDA in niacin will help you stay the course of a healthy mind and body.

Too tired to talk, let alone tango

Doreen drags herself out of bed in the morning, drags herself to work, drags herself home, then drags herself back to bed again at night. Why so tired? While being deficient in any vitamin could slow Doreen down, the most likely candidates are any of four vitamins and three minerals. If Doreen is low in thiamine or riboflavin, some of her crucial energy-producing processes may not work so well, and her body has less energy. In turn, she feels like spending less energy. A deficiency in either B_{12} or folic acid can bring about two fairly rare anemias, both of which produce tiredness. If Doreen lacks chromium, her insulin won't be doing the job it should, her blood sugar will rise, then fall, leaving her exhausted. If she's not getting enough potassium, her muscles won't work as well as they should, and again she'll feel like a slug. But the most probable culprit is iron. Doreen's not eating much in the way of spinach or liver, nor is she taking an iron supplement, and her body's letting her know it with fatigue, one of the most telling signs of inadequate iron.

Vitamin B_6

B_6 is often called "the woman's vitamin," and it is important for women who take birth-control pills. Some women taking oral contraceptives suffer from bouts of depression, and doses of B_6 can be used to alleviate these blues. B_6 therapy may also help control a certain kind of diabetes that pregnant women sometimes develop. If that's not enough, B_6 can help all of us, male or female, by keeping our circulation running freely and strong.

Vitamin B_{12}

B_{12} has the somewhat ill-deserved reputation as a "pep-up" vitamin, the reason being that someone suffering from an acute deficiency of the vitamin, known as pernicious anemia, will suffer from weakness, tiredness, and lethargy and will quickly be re-energized by a shot of B_{12}. Some believe that if you're tired all the time, while you probably don't have pernicious anemia, you might just be slightly low in the vitamin, and making sure you're getting your RDA could possibly bring back a little spring in your step. (Without vitamin therapy, pernicious anemia can lead to yellow skin, loss of appetite and loss of weight, abdominal pain, and other serious symptoms.) B_{12} is of particular concern to *vegans*—strict vegetarians who won't eat any animal products, not even milk or cheese—as the vitamin is found only in animal products. For them, some kind of supplement is usually advisable.

Folic acid

Deficiency in folic acid produces megaloblastic anemia, very similar in its symptoms of weakness, depression, and lethargy to the pernicious anemia brought on by a lack of B_{12} (which is why over-the-counter doses of the vitamin are controlled—taking it could mask a case of pernicious anemia). Although pregnant women run the highest risk of being low in folic acid, a deficiency in it is usually pretty hard to come by. Nevertheless, a slight deficiency might have something to do with dry skin, slow healing, and hair loss. Making sure you're getting your RDA is a small premium to pay for insurance against such a risk. (If you take a folic acid supplement, also take B_{12}.)

Pantothenic acid

Pantothenic acid is a somewhat controversial B-complex vitamin. Key to the performance of our adrenal cortex, it may also have something to do with how well we manage stress—or at least how well rats manage in a stressful situation. One study took rats and tossed them into cold water to sink or swim (about the most stressful situation imaginable for a rat). Those with a little extra pantothenic acid stayed afloat longer than those without. This doesn't necessarily mean pantothenic acid will help you glide through a pressure-filled work day, but it should give you some idea of the vitamin's importance. Because pantothenic acid is found in so many foods, deficiencies are rare, but may occur in those with severe malnutrition or chronic alcoholism.

Because the B vitamins help keep your mind and body running smoothly and because they work best together, plan your intake to cover all of them—don't concentrate on just one or two. Give yourself the benefit of the best that the B-complex group can offer you.

Vitamin C

Scurvy is the most infamous of the deficiences, and its cure, Vitamin C, is the most famous of all vitamins. Recent claims make it out to be the wonder-potion of the age, and while many of these suggestions are intriguing and persuasive, what we already know for sure about the vitamin is astounding.

Because Vitamin C is crucial in keeping your blood vessels strong and your tissues healthy, it's vital in

"SUPERFOODS"—the top ten vitamin and mineral all-stars

These foods are high in a number of different vitamins and minerals. For ideas on how to include these foods in your meals, see Recipes for health, *pages 57-59.*

Food	Vitamins	Minerals
Beef liver	A, B complex, C, biotin, pantothenate	potassium, iron, zinc, selenium
Broccoli	A, C, pantothenate	calcium, iron
Wheat germ	B complex, E	selenium, manganese
Nuts (all sorts)	B complex, E, biotin	phosphorus, zinc
Spinach	A, C	iron
Chicken, white meat	B complex	chromium, iron potassium, zinc
Salmon	B complex, D, E	calcium, potassium
Brewer's yeast	B complex	iron, chromium
Cauliflower	C, biotin, pantothenate	
Cantaloupe	A, C	

Preventing cancer with Vitamin C

Vitamin C may also play a role in preventing cancer caused by nitrates (most commonly found in smoked meats like bacon) by combining with the nitrates and seeing them safely out of the body. Otherwise the nitrates may combine with amines in the stomach, producing nitrosamines that may be cancer-causing.

The sunshine vitamin

Believe it or not, the sun and your skin combine to supply most of your body's Vitamin D requirements. Here's how: *the top layer of your skin contains a substance that, when exposed to the sun's ultraviolet rays, converts to Vitamin D. So the easiest way of preventing Vitamin D deficiency is simply to get out in the sun—your skin will do the rest.*

helping us heal ourselves. People getting the RDA (or a little more, as many feel that 200 mg. is a more optimal level than the present 60 mg. RDA) tend to have their cuts and scrapes heal faster than those who don't. A little extra Vitamin C may aid recovery from infections, burns, and other stresses because these things deplete Vitamin C in the blood.

Vitamin C also helps keep our blood flowing smoothly and free of clots (we only want blood to clot when a wound has to be closed, as clots in the vein can travel to the heart and wreak havoc). This effect on the blood helps prevent heart disease.

Vitamin C has also been shown to be important in how we cope with the stress of temperature extremes. In addition, some studies suggest that Vitamin C acts a little bit like an antihistamine. And, while it won't *cure* a cold (a common misconception), Vitamin C might just keep you from getting one in the first place and might help you feel a little better and get better a little faster if you do get one.

Vitamin D

The "sunshine vitamin" keeps your bones straight and strong. A deficiency in it can lead to rickets among children and *osteomalacia*—a softening of the bones that's potentially crippling—in adults. Its lack is also involved in allowing *osteoporosis* to set in, a condition in which bones lose their calcium and become porous, brittle, and easy to break. If you don't drink milk regularly, you'll need to pay attention to how you get your Vitamin D. (It's particularly abundant in livers and liver oils of many saltwater fish, and also occurs in tuna, salmon, herring, egg yolks, grains, vegetable oils, butter, cheese, and liver.) You'll want to avoid the consequence of insufficient D intake, especially if you're a female over 40.

Of keen interest are some recent Scandinavian studies indicating that people who spend more time in the sun seem to avoid depression, and Vitamin D seems to be the active ingredient in keeping them depression-free. Maybe there's more to the joy we feel while lying on the beach than just being away from work. (The wisdom of a couple of generations ago that everyone needed a daily dose of cod-liver oil is now clear: it's a good source of Vitamin D.) Another good thing about D is that we can build up stores of it, so that people who live in cloudy northern climates can manage for a while without the sun.

Vitamin E

A few years ago, a lot of grand claims were made about this vitamin, and most of them have turned out to be either totally or partially unfounded. Vitamin E is called "the vitamin in search of a deficiency" because no known ill effect accompanies its absence from a person's diet. Although experimenters found that rats with zero Vitamin E were sterile (which is why Vitamin E became incorrectly known as the "sex vitamin"), no similar deficiency effects have been found in humans.

All this doesn't stop E from being important to you. Its greatest role is as an antioxidant. We need oxygen to survive, but just as oxygen can rust, or oxidize, metal, so it can do damage in our bodies by oxidizing and spoiling the vital fat in our cells. Fortunately, antioxidants block this process, and Vitamin E is one of the most effective antioxidants.

Another great chore of E is to help manage the level of cholesterol in your blood. While cholesterol is vital and we all need some of it, too much can threaten the health of our arteries, introducing the risk of atherosclerosis and heart disease. Vitamin E, however, is associated with raising the level of a certain kind of cholesterol—a "safe" cholesterol—in our blood that actually lowers the risk of heart disease.

Other attributes include E's application as an effective part of a skin moisturizer, and the fact that many people claim it can heal cuts and burns. Because it's an antioxidant, E does help reduce scarring during healing.

Symptoms

Not every ill is attributable solely to a vitamin or mineral deficiency—dry skin, hair loss, fatigue, brittle nails, or bleeding gums can be caused by any number of different ailments, some more or less serious than others. If you have any of the symptoms mentioned anywhere in this chapter or throughout the book, go see your doctor. He or she will be able to tell if your inability to see well at night is because you haven't been eating your carrots or if it's due to something else. Your concern for your diet and your intake of vitamins and minerals should be just one part of your overall interest in your health.

Calcium

Calcium works hand in hand with Vitamin D as the guardian of the health of your bones, and a deficiency in this mineral can arise quite easily. Making sure you're getting your calcium—and a lot of people aren't, especially women and the elderly—will help ward off osteoporosis and keep your bones strong. Exercise is also important, as the repeated pressure on your bones from running, walking, bicycling, or other aerobic exercise (but not swimming, as it doesn't cause any pressure on your bones) helps your bones absorb calcium.

Vitamin E and atherosclerosis

Without vitamin E to manage the cholesterol level in your blood, you could develop atherosclerosis. Here's how:

Atherosclerosis begins when an injury or other event makes the artery's wall permeable to cholesterol and other fatty substances. When these substances work their way into the walls, they produce a fatty streak. Eventually, a fibrous plaque forms and slows the blood flow through the artery. Finally, the plaque can calcify or rupture and may cause thrombosis and almost totally block the artery.

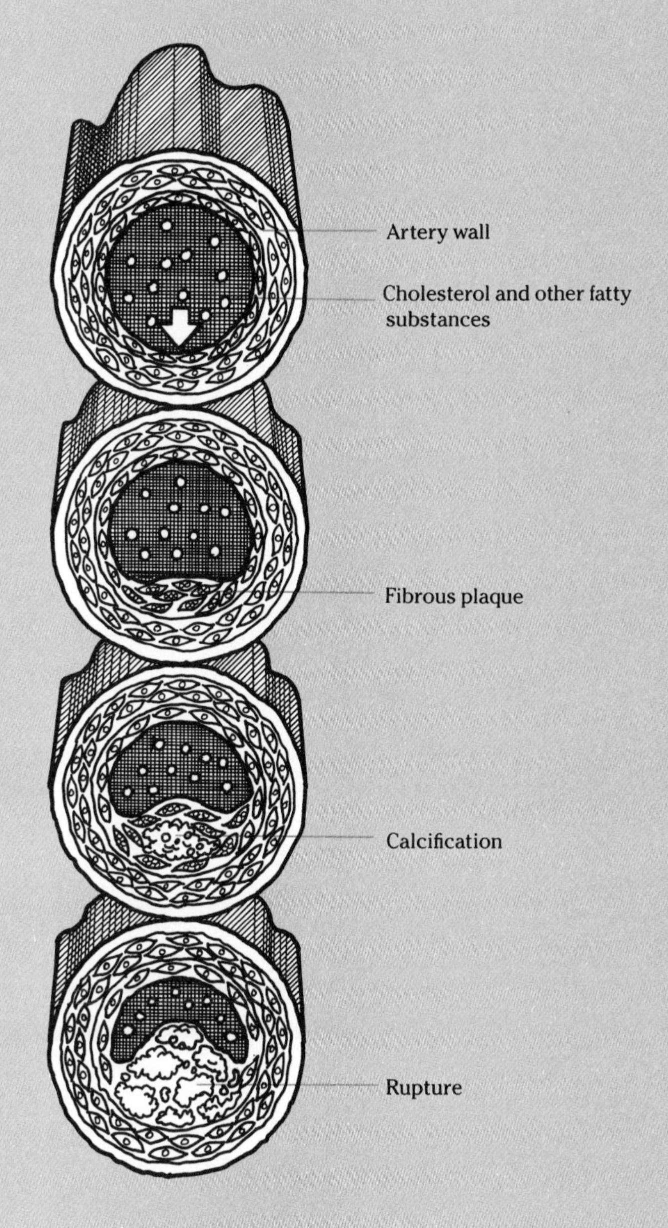

Try calcium for a good night's sleep

Calcium is known as nature's tranquilizer for its role in calming people and helping them sleep and cope with stress. So if you suffer from insomnia or stress, try relaxing with a calcium-rich glass of warm milk, a few slices of Swiss cheese, a sardine sandwich, or a dish of yogurt or ice cream.

Some antacid tablets contain up to 500 mg. of calcium carbonate. Although this is an unexpected source of calcium, those who suffer from indigestion may want to count this calcium as part of their daily intake.

Calcium must usually be accompanied by Vitamin D for it to be absorbed properly. Dolomite, however, is a natural form that can be absorbed without Vitamin D. Bonemeal, another natural form, is, however, harder to absorb than the synthetic forms of calcium such as calcium gluconate, carbonate, and lactate. Also, the synthetic forms don't contain any lead while the natural forms can.

The other natural partner with calcium is magnesium. They work together for improved cardiovascular health. In the case of magnesium alone, there's evidence that in areas where magnesium intake is high, there's a reduction in the incidence of surprise heart attacks.

Chromium

Another mineral that may have something to do with preventing heart attacks is chromium. People who die of heart disease have been shown to have less chromium in their aorta (the heart's major artery) than those who die from other causes. Chromium seems to be especially adept at preventing blood clots, which may be why it helps guard against heart disease.

Too much of a good thing

Chromium's an important mineral for several reasons. It's necessary for glucose metabolism and may prevent heart attacks. But in large amounts, chromium can cause toxicity. Certain workers can be exposed to high levels of chromium on the job when they inhale or touch it. Industrial workers at the highest risk may include those in:

- *Abrasives manufacturing*
- *Cement manufacturing*
- *Diesel locomotive repair*
- *Electroplating*
- *Explosive manufacturing*
- *Furniture polishing*
- *Fur processing*

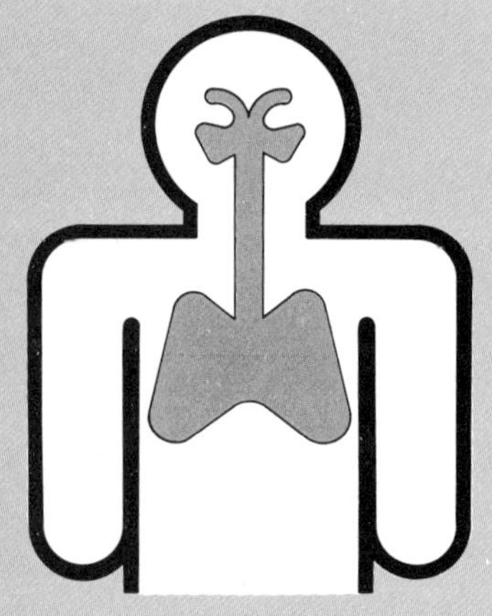

- *Glassmaking*
- *Jewelry making*
- *Metal cleaning*
- *Oil drilling*
- *Photography*
- *Textile dyeing*
- *Wood preservative manufacturing*

Two ways to increase iron absorption

One trick: if you take Vitamin C with your iron-rich foods, your absorption of iron can be boosted up to ten times normal. Another trick: cook tomato-based dishes in an iron skillet or Dutch oven. Acidic foods will leach some iron out of the pot.

Chromium also may be good for your heart because of its tie to insulin. High levels of insulin in the blood (caused because the insulin that's there isn't working efficiently, so your pancreas sends out more to do the job) may have something to do with hardening of the arteries and heart disease. Indeed, insulin-related heart disease is the number-one killer of diabetics, who might benefit from adequate chromium.

On a less dramatic level, chromium may also have something to do with the proper development of your teeth.

Iron

Hemoglobin is the part of the red blood cell that carries iron throughout your body. Without adequate iron, your body slows down. The symptoms of iron-deficiency anemia make for a long list: weakness, dizzy spells, apathy, hair loss, fainting, poor appetite, brittle nails. The symptoms, although many, aren't the sort that make you think of a mineral deficiency: there are a dozen reasons why you might be tired, for example, so a deficiency can often go unnoticed for a time. At highest risk are growing children and women. So if you're feeling a little too tired some of the time, a lack of iron just may be the culprit. In any event, make a habit of eating iron-rich food.

Potassium

Potassium works in a very careful balancing act with sodium, which, when tipped in favor of sodium, can lead to higher blood pressure. You'll benefit from keeping your sodium intake down and your potassium intake in proportion (about 2 to 1 in favor of potassium). Of course, potassium does more than just balance with sodium. It also works with your muscles, keeping them healthy. If you exercise, watch your potassium (especially if it's hot because you can sweat it out fast) —your muscles can stiffen up if you don't have it.

Zinc

This mineral is involved in a wide variety of metabolic processes. It helps control growth, sexual development, wound healing, and maintenance of skin, hair, nails, and mucous membranes. The biggest beneficiary of zinc's powers is your skin. It's been used for ages as the ingredient in calamine lotion, soothing itchy skin. We get most of our zinc from meat, eggs,

Beware of vitamin and mineral fads

In recent years, marketers have touted such things as zinc and vitamin E as cures for everything from acne to impotence. These claims are often based on inconclusive research or even on stories from people who believe their ailments were cured when they took this vitamin or that mineral.

When you hear such claims and you're tempted to try something new, be sure to do a little research of your own first. And if the claims still sound suspicious to you, ask your doctor for more information.

Healing the hurts

Randy is a bike rider who tends to fall down, bump into things, and generally get a lot of cuts and scrapes. But his mother doesn't mind, because Randy's cuts heal fast, and he's a good kid. In fact, it's because he's a good kid that his cuts heal fast. Randy actually eats his peas and carrots, both of which are high in Vitamin A, a vitamin that helps speed the healing process. Randy also helps himself by drinking a couple of glasses of orange juice a day, and the Vitamin C in the juice also helps tissues grow and skin heal quickly. And he even eats liver, high not only in A, but in the B-complex vitamins and zinc, all of which also help heal hurts faster. Now, if he just wouldn't ride his bike so fast...

liver, and seafood, although vegetarians can find a more than adequate supply in whole grains, nuts, and beans.

Other minerals

Other minerals—copper, fluorine, iodine, phosphorus—are crucial to the proper functioning of your body and even have some therapeutic value, such as fluorine, which protects your teeth. However, most of these minerals are so prevalent in our diet—so much so that in some cases we might worry about getting too much rather than too little—that we need have no concern about getting enough.

Each of these minerals has an important role to play:

• Copper helps the body use iron properly and is essential to the manufacture of hemoglobin and blood cells in the bone marrow. Most people can get enough copper from the foods they eat, especially if they include liver, shellfish, nuts, and dried beans in their diets.

• Fluorine exists in almost all soil, water, plants, and animals. And in many places, fluorine is added to the water supply. It's essential for dental health and also helps bones develop normally.

• Iodine is a part of thyroxine—a thyroid hormone—which controls the body's metabolism. Good sources of iodine are seafoods and iodized salt.

• Phosphorus teams up with calcium to promote bone growth, strength, and maintenance. It also takes part in reactions that produce energy, especially those involved with muscle contractions. Phosphorus deficiency is unusual, because phosphorus is found in most foods.

Other minerals, such as selenium, silicon, and manganese, may have therapeutic value, but the evidence with them is not yet all in.

Recipes for health

By combining recipes, you could come up with a dinner menu that should please even the most discerning palate. It will also please the vitamin needs of your body.

- Before-dinner snack: *Bowls of various nuts, in and out of shell.*
- Hors d'oeuvres: *Cheese and Vegetable Dip with vegetable sticks and crackers.*
- Salad: *Tossed green-leaf lettuce with an olive oil, red wine vinegar, and Dijon mustard dressing.*
- Main Dish: *Liver with Herbs or Broiled Salmon with Dill.*
- Vegetables: *Carrot Strips with Snow Peas, Baked Potatoes Plus*
- Dessert: *Fruit Salad*

This menu is just one of many possibilities. A couple of good cookbooks, some attention to choosing vitamin- and mineral-rich foods, a little individual imagination, and you'll command healthful and delicious menus.

Carrot strips and snow peas

3 large carrots
1/4 pound snow peas
2 tablespoons butter or vegetable oil
2 tablespoons raw sesame seeds
1/2 teaspoon chopped garlic
1 tablespoon soy sauce
2 tablespoons chopped green onions or chives

This recipe for a dinner vegetable dish made with carrots and snow peas is quite high in Vitamin A.

1. Wash the carrots and trim off the ends. Then cut the carrots into thin strips about 1 1/2 inches long. Trim the ends off the snow peas and slice them into strips about 1/4 inch wide.

2. Drop the carrots into boiling water. Cover and simmer for four minutes. Then add the snow peas. Stir and simmer for another two minutes; then drain.

3. Melt the butter in a frying pan and add raw sesame seeds, stir-frying the seeds until they're light brown (a minute or two). Then add the garlic, carrots, snow peas, soy sauce, and chopped green onions. Stir-fry for another minute, then serve.

Makes six servings.

Continued

Recipes for health *(continued)*

Liver and herbs

- 1½ pounds calves' liver, in eight thin slices
- pepper to taste
- ¼ cup flour
- 2 tablespoons corn, vegetable, or peanut oil
- 6 tablespoons butter
- 2 tablespoons finely chopped shallots
- 1 tablespoon red wine vinegar
- 2 tablespoons finely chopped parsley
- 2 tablespoons finely chopped chives
- 1 teaspoon finely chopped tarragon

Beef liver, although high in calories and cholesterol, is an excellent source of Vitamin A, most of the B vitamins, chromium, zinc, and iron. For every person who hates liver you'll find another who loves it. This recipe might convert a few haters into lovers.

1. Sprinkle both sides of the liver slices with pepper and flour.

2. Heat the oil in a large frying pan and cook the liver until nicely brown on both sides (1 minute or longer each side, depending on thickness).

3. Transfer the cooked slices to a warm platter and keep warm.

4. Wipe the pan clean, then heat the butter until it's melted and browning. Add the shallots and vinegar and cook a few seconds. Pour this brown butter mixture over the liver, then sprinkle with the remaining herbs and serve.

Makes four servings.

Fruit salad

Fruit salad makes for an excellent dessert. It's also good just to have around in the refrigerator as a snack. And it's very simple to make. Just take an assortment of fruits, chop them up into bite-size chunks, and mix them together in a bowl. The best bets are oranges, apples, strawberries, blueberries, grapefruit, and the like, all of which are high in Vitamin C. Chunks of watermelon will give you Vitamin A, and small scoops of canteloupe will provide high quantities of both A and C. Other welcome additions are seedless grapes, slices of kiwi for an exotic touch, and chunks of banana and pineapple to provide a little added sweetness. Serve chilled.

Salmon with dill

- 4 salmon steaks, 6 ounces each, boneless
- pepper to taste
- 4 tablespoons chopped fresh dill
- 1 tablespoon olive oil
- 2 tablespoons fresh lemon juice

As an alternative to liver as an entree, here's a salmon dish high in the B-complex vitamins and very high in Vitamin D. It's delicious, easy to prepare, and no more expensive than most cuts of meat.

1. Pepper the salmon, then sprinkle it with dill.

2. Stir the olive oil and lemon juice together and pour this mixture over the salmon. Cover the salmon and marinate it in the refrigerator for two hours.

3. Preheat the broiler, and broil the salmon, skin-side down, about four inches from the heat for not much more than five minutes. Test the fish by flaking it with a fork. It should be cooked but still moist.

Makes four servings.

A bowl full of nuts

It's as simple as that. The best source of Vitamin E (and a good source of zinc, too) is almost any kind of nut. Almost any mixture will do. A good bet is to include almonds, pecans, hazelnuts, peanuts (not technically nuts!), walnuts, and brazil nuts (these last two are also good sources of magnesium). You can either present them in their shell with a nutcracker on the side, or you can shell them beforehand. Nuts are also high in protein and make an excellent snack food. Just eat them while they're fresh, because their oils can turn rancid, which will destroy Vitamin E.

Cheese and vegetable dip

1 pound sharp cheddar cheese
1 bunch broccoli
½ cup whole milk
1 can cream of mushroom soup

The greatest food source of calcium is cheese. On a platter, with some crackers and a few slices of apple, cheese can make a wonderful before- or after-dinner snack. Below is a recipe for a very simple cheddar cheese dip.

1. Grate the cheese.

2. Chop the broccoli into small bits, using primarily the flowerettes.

3. Put the milk into a saucepan, heat, and add the cheese. Stir until melted and liquid. Add more milk if necessary, until the mixture is the consistency of heavy cream.

*4. Add the broccoli and the can of cream of mushroom soup (*do not *add the milk or water that the soup directions call for).*

5. Heat through, over low heat, about ten minutes. Serve hot or cold with crackers and raw vegetables for dipping.

Makes four servings.

Baked potatoes plus

Potatoes are one of the best food sources of potassium. Baking them is perhaps the easiest way to prepare them, and with a little added effort and some imagination you can make them very exciting. All it requires is baking (a medium to large Idaho at 350° needs a little under an hour). Using oven mitts to protect your hands, open each potato and scoop out the insides. Put this in a mixing bowl and let your imagination and taste buds go to work. Mix in grated cheddar cheese, or sour cream, or yogurt or fresh chives, dill, or any combination. Then take the mixture, stuff it back into the potato skins, and put the whole thing back in the oven to heat through.

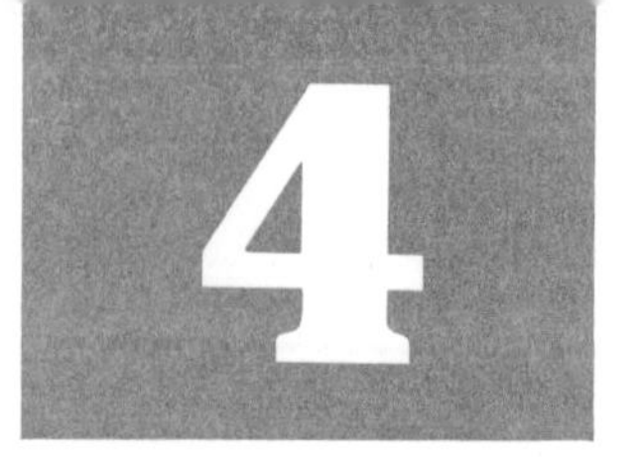

Special needs of women

The woman's vitamin

There's some indication that B_6, already known as the "woman's vitamin," may help alleviate some of the debilitating symptoms of PMS—premenstrual syndrome—suffered by some women.

Estrogen and vitamins

Estrogen—a hormone that occurs naturally in humans and animals—is also produced synthetically and used as drug therapy to help bring about certain body changes. If your doctor prescribes estrogen therapy for you, you'll need to take more Vitamins C and B_6 as well, because estrogen increases the body's need for these vitamins. Here are some common reasons why women use estrogen therapy:

- *as replacement therapy, if the body isn't producing enough estrogen on its own*
- *to treat vaginal infection or vulvar rash, caused by chronic estrogen deficiency*
- *to start menstrual periods and relieve amenorrhea—the absence of menstruation*
- *to relieve breast engorgement after giving birth*
- *to stop growth of certain types of cancerous tumors*
- *as a contraceptive (along with progestogen)*
- *to help prevent osteoporosis, used along with calcium.*

Women have special vitamin and mineral needs throughout their lives—and at different times of their lives. When a woman starts menstruating, her iron needs increase. Women who take oral contraceptives often have reduced blood levels of thiamine, riboflavin, B_6, B_{12}, folic acid, and Vitamin C. Some pregnant or breast-feeding women need vitamin and mineral supplements to meet their nutritional needs. And after menopause, when estrogen levels decline, women need extra Vitamin D and calcium to keep their bones healthy and strong.

Iron and calcium

All women should make sure they're getting enough iron and calcium, for they're the two most common deficiencies among women. The big trouble with iron is that while most adults generally lose 1 to 2 mg. of it every day, we absorb only about one-tenth of what we take in—which is why the RDA is set at 18 mg. for adults: that's the least amount we need to make sure we're replacing the iron we're losing. But women lose more still. The most direct loss of iron in women happens every month during their menstrual blood loss, and they have to make sure they're getting extra iron to make up for that. Women with heavy menstrual bleeding will lose even more iron, and therefore require even more new iron.

The other great deficiency in women is calcium. Women's absorption of the mineral starts to taper off about the time they reach 20, and their bones actually start to get drained of it starting at age 25. That's right—this deficiency, most often associated with the elderly, begins just a few years after college. When calcium is insufficient, the body leeches it from the bones. The bones gradually become porous, brittle, easy to fracture. This condition is known as osteoporosis. Women of all ages should make sure they're getting enough calcium—1,000 mg. a day up to menopause, 1,200 mg. a day thereafter—as well as Vitamin D, which is calcium's partner in guarding the health of bones. They should also be sure to exercise regularly because it's pressure on the bones—from jogging, walk-

Eating for two

When you're pregnant or breast-feeding, you're truly eating for two. That doesn't mean you should eat twice as much as you normally do. In fact, most women need only about 15% more calories during pregnancy or while breast-feeding. But eating for two does mean you should increase your intake of vitamins and minerals to make sure both you and your baby get enough. Most doctors prescribe multivitamin and mineral supplements during this time, as added insurance to keep mother and baby properly nourished. To understand your increased nutritional needs, see the U.S. Recommended Daily Allowances (U.S. RDAs) for pregnant and breast-feeding women on page 25.

ing, bicycling, or any aerobic exercise (except swimming)—that causes the calcium to be set in and remain in the bones.

Contraceptives

Women taking oral contraceptives also have their own special nutritional needs. These are caused by what contraceptives are and what they do. Oral contraceptives are essentially hormones—estrogen, usually—that throw off a woman's hormonal balance, stopping the release of any eggs from the ovaries. Estrogens can cause deficiencies of certain vitamins. They remove folic acid from the blood, deplete stores of Vitamin C, and, as they are detoxified by the liver, raise requirements for one of the liver's workhorses, riboflavin. The most blatant contraceptive-induced deficiency is B_6, a lack of which can bring on depression in some women; this depression can be lifted simply by taking supplements of the vitamin.

Pregnancy

For several reasons, pregnant women may need more of certain vitamins and minerals. The old adage that mothers-to-be are "eating for two" is quite true when it comes to vitamin and mineral requirements. There are separate RDA levels for many vitamins and minerals for pregnant women simply because the growth and nurturing of the fetus demands extra nutrients. Pregnant women often have low levels of thiamine, biotin, and pantothenate (although whether they're low in these B vitamins because their bodies aren't absorbing them as well, are flushing them out faster, or are using more of them isn't known). Pregnant women should make very sure they're getting at least their RDA in these three essential Bs.

How your diet affects your baby

When you're pregnant, the amount of blood circulating in your body must increase by 50 to 60 percent to nourish the placenta, the organ that develops inside the uterus and functions as your link with the fetus. The food you eat allows your blood volume to increase and provides the placenta with the nutrients it needs to keep healthy. Together, your blood and the placenta serve as the transport medium for the nutrients and oxygen that pass from you into the fetus, and the waste products that pass from the fetus to you. Any food you eat or drug you take may cross the placenta and enter the fetal circulation. That's why you need to eat right during pregnancy and to follow your doctor's advice about taking over-the-counter and prescription drugs—including vitamin and mineral pills.

Adjusting the four food groups

If you're pregnant, the best way to satisfy your own and your baby's nutritional needs is to eat a wide variety of high-quality foods from the four major food groups. Because you're pregnant, you'll need to help yourself to more daily servings of foods from certain food groups—milk and milk products, for example. That way, you'll be more likely to get the right amount of vitamins and minerals you need. Here's what you need each day:

Food group	Number of daily servings
Milk and milk products	4
Protein-rich foods	2-3
Fruits and vegetables	4-6
Grains	4-5

Other vitamins and minerals have more specific roles during pregnancy, and their presence or absence can have a more obvious effect. The two most common deficiencies during pregnancy are iron and folic acid. Throughout its growth, the fetus will need, in total, roughly 300 to 500 mg. of iron. With the RDA set at 18 mg. for pregnant women, and with a total of nine months for the fetus to get its requirement, no problem should arise. But women—pregnant or not—have a hard enough time just getting their own RDA, let alone enough for two, so an iron supplement during pregnancy is likely to be necessary.

Folic acid deficiency, just as common as a lack of iron, can get quite serious. Because this vitamin plays a key role in the growth and development of tissues, a lack of it can spell trouble, leading to possible birth defects. And a lack of folic acid doesn't just cause problems for the fetus, but for the mother as well. Low levels of this vitamin have been associated with "restless leg syndrome," which gives pregnant women muscle cramps and insomnia. Given adequate folic acid, the problem can clear up. Furthermore, the postpartum depression that some women suffer may also be caused by a folic acid deficiency.

Pregnant women also have higher needs for calcium and Vitamin D, not only to keep their own bones healthy and strong, but to start their babies' bones on the right path as well. (The needs will continue through breast-feeding.) Requirements for Vitamin C are also high during pregnancy, and even higher while the mother is breast-feeding since the vitamin is necessary to prevent scurvy in the infant. Another vitamin that should be monitored during pregnancy is B_{12}. Some children are born with birth defects caused by pernicious anemia—a lack of B_{12}. If this deficiency is diagnosed well before birth with some of the more modern techniques of prenatal care, B_{12} supplements given the mother will eliminate the risk of pernicious anemic birth defects.

Menopause

With both calcium and Vitamin D, women seem to need more as they get older. Yet they also eat less cheese and drink less milk, partly because these foods are high in calories, partly because they're hard to digest. Thus, many women pass up the two food sources in which calcium and Vitamin D are most abundant. This makes supplementation necessary for older women.

Why osteoporosis happens

When the body uses up its store of calcium, osteoporosis—the most common chronic health problem facing women over age 45—can result. To help prevent osteoporosis, you need to understand what makes it occur.

Normally, a group of hormones works to keep a constant level of calcium in your bloodstream, so calcium can travel to all the tissues that need it. If your diet doesn't supply enough calcium, these hormones remove some from your bones, where 90% of your body's calcium supply is stored. Over time, this depletes the bones' calcium store, making them porous, brittle, and easily broken: osteoporosis. If osteoporosis isn't corrected, the spinal vertebrae begin to collapse, eventually leading to an abnormal curvature of the spine and "dowager's hump."

Here's how to help keep your body from using up calcium faster than you can replace it:

- *Get enough calcium in your diet. Make sure you have three servings of milk products every day, or take the recommended amount of calcium supplements.*
- *Avoid foods that are high in phosphorus. The more phosphorus-rich foods you eat—for example, meat, carbonated beverages, and processed foods—the less calcium your body absorbs, because phosphorus competes with calcium for absorption.*
- *Keep active, and exercise regularly. Inactivity speeds up the loss of calcium and results in bone loss. On the positive side, exercise stimulates bone growth by increasing tension on bones and ligaments.*

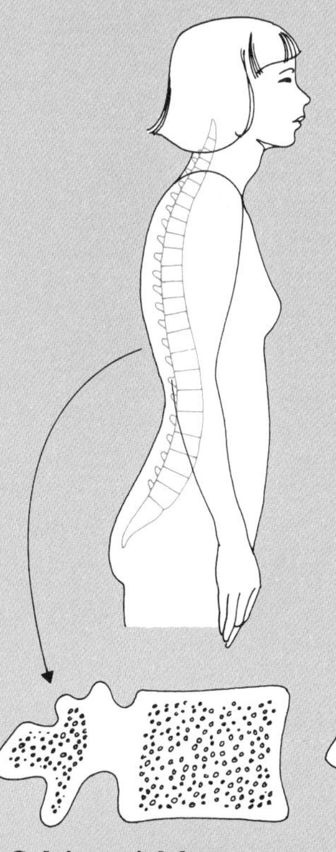

Calcium-rich bones produce a normal, strong spine.

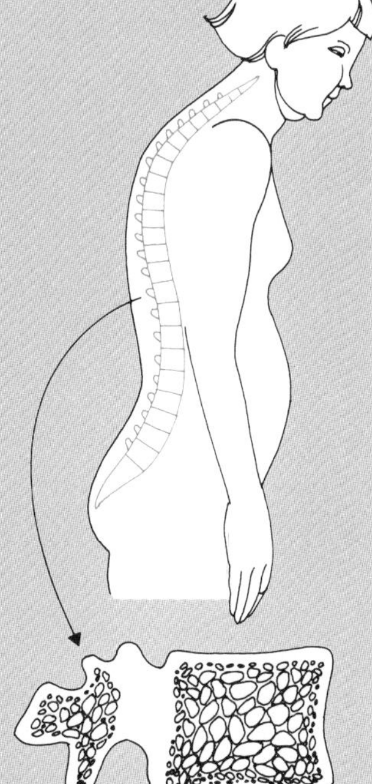

Calcium-poor bones cause osteoporosis and abnormal spine curvature.

5 Special needs of the elderly

How aging affects body composition

As you get older, your body's composition changes and you need less food. (You may also be less active.)

Lean body mass usually decreases and the percentage of body fat usually increases (unless you maintain a youthful level of exercise). Thus you're "fatter" at age 75 than you were at age 20, even if you weigh the same.

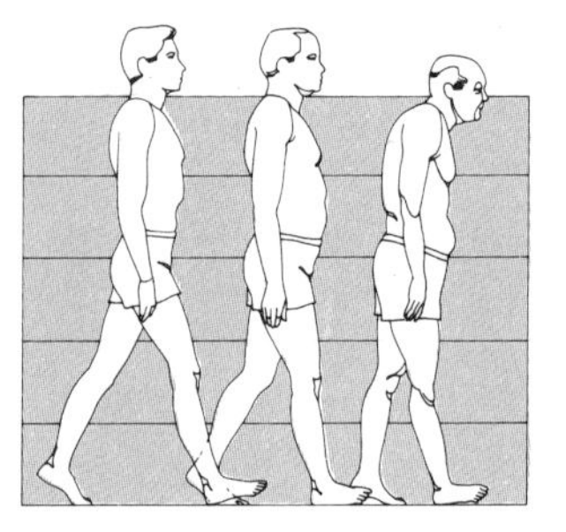

People live longer than they used to. This increase in life expectancy is the result in large part of improved health care—and improved nutrition. A healthy diet can help you live a longer life, and the need for proper nutrition doesn't diminish as you grow older.

Unfortunately, many elderly people don't get enough vitamins and minerals in their diet. Recent surveys report disturbing figures: for example, 60 percent of the elderly may be deficient in folic acid, 55 percent in B_6, and 34 percent in thiamine.

The elderly are prone to vitamin and mineral deficiencies for two reasons: they're simply not getting enough, and they have higher requirements than they had when they were younger.

Why aren't the elderly getting enough vitamins and minerals? Some elderly people suffer the depleting effects of restrictive diets, disease, and drugs. What's more, as our bodies age, their ability to digest and absorb nutrients decreases. Poverty, poor teeth, and loneliness can also have effects on the amount of food—and vitamins and minerals—many elderly people eat.

The older you get, the less food—fuel—your body needs. Unfortunately, there's no accompanying drop in your body's requirement for nutrients. Thus, while the elderly may require less food, they still need roughly the same amount of vitamins and minerals as when they were younger. Indeed, their requirements for some vitamins and minerals can increase.

Thiamine

More and more evidence suggests that senior citizens in our society are the most vitamin and mineral needy. What vitamins and minerals are they low in? Thiamine is one. While thiamine deficiencies in the elderly may only infrequently get to the extreme stage of beriberi, even mild deficiencies can have a profound effect. One of the great concerns for the well-being of the elderly concerns their mental health, and severe deficiencies in thiamine can produce impaired mental faculties. Since a decrease in the level of the vitamin can bring on symptoms that may mimic other mental problems,

Which form of calcium

You can fight osteoporosis with calcium supplementation, but calcium supplements aren't all the same. Some forms are less readily absorbed by the body than others.

Be sure to ask your doctor about the best form of calcium supplement for you. Whichever he suggests, he'll probably recommend that you take any calcium supplement with meals to facilitate normal absorption.

a "dotty old aunt" really may not be dotty at all but just may not be getting the amount of thiamine in her diet that she needs.

Vitamin C and iron

The elderly can be low in B_6 and folic acid. They may also be deficient in another B-complex vitamin, biotin. Two other commonly missing nutrients are Vitamin C and iron (even though their requirements for iron are less than when they were younger, the elderly still might not get even that). Perhaps because many elderly people wear dentures, they don't want to chomp down on the firmer, harder fruits and vegetables that are high in Vitamin C. Iron is high in several of nature's most disliked foods—such as liver and spinach—and it's hard to convince someone who hasn't liked or eaten those foods for 60 years that he or she should start now.

Vitamins and medicines

Another reason the elderly might not be getting all the vitamins and minerals they need is that the medicines they often have to take can deplete certain nutrients. One example of this is mineral oil, which is widely used as a laxative. Unfortunately, mineral oil can block the absorption of all the fat-soluble vitamins, A, D, and E, as well as interfere with the absorption of minerals and proteins.

Changing needs

The other main reason why the elderly are low in certain vitamins and minerals is that some of their requirements go up as they get older. Such is the case with calcium. The older we get, the less well our bodies absorb calcium. When calcium intake is insufficient, our bodies drain calcium from our bones. Our bones gradually become porous and brittle, resulting in osteoporosis. The older we get, the more we should take of this mineral, and along with it some Vitamin D and Vitamin C, which also keep our bones strong.

Ultimately, the elderly have to take special care of themselves with what they eat. Some argue that there's little point in changing your eating habits at age 70. On the other hand, a better diet can make you feel better and improve the quality of your life. Choose your food carefully. If eating properly is impossible, consider taking some form of supplement, with special emphasis on the B complex, Vitamin C, Vitamin D, and essential minerals, to cover all the bases.

Solving a problem

Because of skin changes, older skin is less able to synthesize Vitamin D from sunlight. Older people who can drink fortified milk should do so. Others can use fish-liver oil.

Adapting a diet to your needs

Sometimes physical problems—such as ill-fitting dentures, sore gums, constipation, gas, diarrhea, or a special diet—can make eating unpleasant. The following tips will help you deal with these problems.

- Are you having difficulty chewing? If so, try including softer foods in your diet; for example, such dairy products as cottage cheese or yogurt; casseroles made with finely ground meat or cheese; canned or very soft fruits, such as bananas; steamed fruits and vegetables that can be chopped or mashed; and cooked cereals, such as oatmeal.

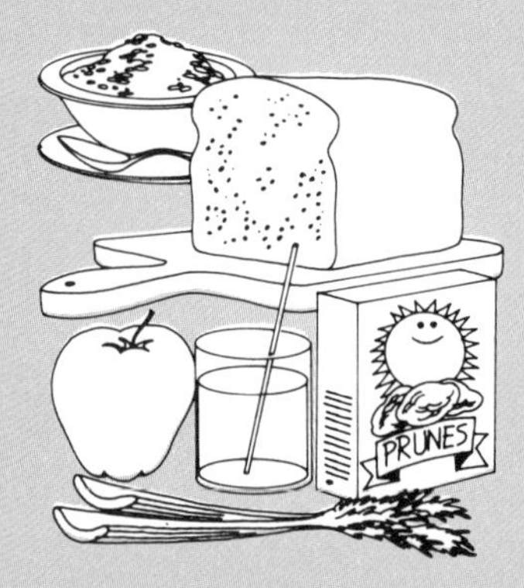

- To help prevent constipation, be sure to include high-fiber foods in your diet. Select from whole grain breads and cereals, cooked or raw fruits or vegetables, prunes in any form, or juice. Also, drink at least 8 full glasses of water daily. Avoid using laxatives, unless ordered by your doctor. And never take mineral oil, as it depletes the body's Vitamin A supply.
- Gas is usually caused by swallowing air while eating rapidly, gulping liquids, chewing gum, or sucking hard candy. (A food that you lack enzymes to digest can also cause gas.) If you seem prone to gas, try to eat and drink slowly and avoid chewing gum and eating hard candy. Remember to sit up straight when eating, and try eating small meals frequently. Also, avoid gas-producing foods and beverages, such as onions, beans, cabbage, and beer.
- Do you experience painful cramps when you drink milk or eat other milk products? If you do, your body may not produce enough of the digestive enzyme lactase. This enzyme breaks the milk sugar lactose into smaller products during digestion. If you can't drink whole milk, you may find that you can comfortably consume lactose-free milk or such fermented milk products as buttermilk, yogurt, and cheese.
- Do you find you don't have much interest in food? Try using herbs, spices, and lemon juice to flavor your foods. Take a cooking class to learn new food preparation techniques. Also, dish out small portions for yourself on a small-sized plate rather than heaping your plate with food you don't really want. Garnish your plate attractively with parsley, or orange or lemon slices. Make a special effort to make your place setting appealing, using attractive placemats, napkins, and tableware. You may find a glass of wine will increase your appetite.
- If you eat alone and don't enjoy it, try eating while you watch the news or another television show or read or listen to music. Or eat outside in good weather.

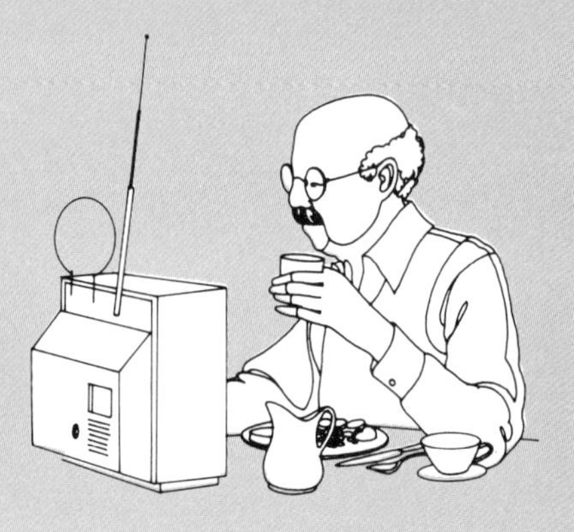

6 Special needs of infants and children

Feeding your child

If you decide to bottle-feed your infant, learn what to look for in a formula. It's good that straight cow's milk isn't used much as formula anymore since it does not make a great formula. It's a poor source of both Vitamin C and copper. You'll want those nutrients along with Vitamin B_6 and iron in your baby's formula.

When you start buying baby foods, read the nutritional labels. For the most part you'll find that fruits will give a good deal of Vitamin C, some Vitamin A, and very little iron or protein. The vegetables, especially strained carrots and creamed spinach, are high in Vitamin A and medium in protein, iron, and Vitamin C. Meats and fish are highest in protein and Vitamin A and lower in Vitamin C and iron. The cereal preparations are the highest source of iron but lowest in the other nutrients. You also want to be on the lookout for added sugar (in all its forms, including corn syrup and honey), salt, starches, and preservatives. The best bet are the ones with no additives (added for the mother's taste buds anyway, not the infant's), and most major brands now provide that alternative. The freeze-dried baby foods are generally lower in additives, but they too should be checked.

Our nutritional needs begin before we're born. Some fetuses can develop a deficiency in B_{12}, and if it's not diagnosed, the pernicious anemia that accompanies it can cause birth defects. If the deficiency is diagnosed, a B_{12} shot given to the mother can eliminate the problem. Similarly, biotin can be low in some newborn babies, bringing on such deficiency symptoms as scaly skin. This too can be prevented if the mother makes sure she's getting all the biotin she and her baby need.

Shortly after birth we receive our first supplement—Vitamin K. This vitamin is crucial to our blood's ability to coagulate. Without it, our blood would be unable to clot and stop the bleeding when we cut ourselves. For almost all of us, the shot of K we get after birth is likely to be the only supplement of that vitamin we'll ever receive. Normally, we produce it ourselves from bacteria in our colon, but newborn babies don't have much in the way of bacteria to do the job at the beginning, and so the shot of K sees them through until their own factories are working.

Breast-feeding versus bottle-feeding

It's after birth, during the breast-feeding stage, that the vitamin and mineral needs of the infant first really become apparent. There has been a long-running argument over the various pros and cons of breast-feeding and bottle-feeding. While there is no one answer for everyone, both methods have their special nutritional concerns. Biotin deficiency among infants occurs most often when they are breast-fed, so mothers opting for that method must make sure they're getting enough of that B-complex vitamin. If bottle-feeding is the chosen method, the mother must make sure the formula contains both B_6 and iron—and good amounts of them, as even some formulas supposedly "fortified" with iron have been found lacking. They should also be aware that breast-feeding passes along antibodies to the infant, and bottle-feeding can't. Also, mothers using cow's milk to nurse their infant should be aware that it is a poor source of Vitamin C and copper. With infants, even a mild deficiency of Vitamin C can result in a minor form of scurvy. As for copper—a

Just for the taste of it

The reason baby foods contain additives like monosodium glutamate (MSG), salt, and sugar is so they won't taste so bland—not to the babies, but to their mothers, who often taste what they feed their infants. The babies aren't bothered by blandness, but they're not the ones who buy the food. Manufacturers are afraid that mothers won't buy their product again if they don't like the taste of it.

mineral that adults are only rarely deficient in—when it's missing in children it can hamper the proper development of bones and teeth and can lead to a loss of the sense of taste.

Baby foods

After milk or formula, the next type of food for babies is usually some sort of baby food. If you don't prepare your own baby foods, read the labels of those you buy to check what percentages of the RDA the foods provide. Go for the ones without added salt, sugar, starches, and preservatives.

As children grow, their nutritional needs are the same or greater than those of adults. Thoughtful diet planning is crucial in these years, for while some children will eat almost anything, others can be quite finicky and you'll need to plan menus carefully to meet all dietary needs. Growing up, we were all told to drink our milk, and it's good that we drank it. Not only is milk an excellent source of protein, but two of the most vital nutrients in a child's diet, calcium and Vitamin D, are found in milk, and they're crucial in insuring the proper growth and development of bones and teeth.

Children's nutritional needs

As a child ages, his Recommended Daily Allowance (RDA) for many vitamins and minerals changes. For instance, the RDA of vitamin A is 1,500 International

Making your own baby food

When you make your own baby food, you can control exactly what goes into it. You can make sure that your child gets his vitamins and minerals, and you can protect him from getting additives and traces of food that he may be sensitive to. Make most baby food in a blender or cook it to a soft consistency. Here are two recipes that you may want to try.

Fruit with cottage cheese

½ cup raw or cooked fresh fruit
½ cup cottage cheese
4 to 6 tablespoons orange juice

Blend all ingredients together until smooth. Serve cool.

Vegetable soup

¼ cup pureed cooked vegetables
1 tablespoon margarine or butter
1 tablespoon whole wheat flour
¼ cup water, broth, or milk

Mix ingredients in a sauce pan and stir until warm.

Adapted from Vicky Lansky, *Feed Me, I'm Yours,* Meadowbrook Press, Deephaven, Minn., 1974.

A spoonful of sugar

"A spoonful of sugar helps the medicine go down"—this Mary Poppins *song line describes exactly why children's chewable vitamins are sweet—so that the kids will eat them without complaint. The trouble is, they can taste so good that children may be tempted to eat them like candy, which can be dangerous. Keep all medicines (even the vitamins children are supposed to take) out of sight and out of reach of children, preferably in childproof containers.*

Units (I.U.) for an infant, 2,500 I.U. for a toddler, and 5,000 I.U. for a child over age 4. (See the *U.S. Recommended Daily Allowances* chart on page 25.) By the time a child reaches age 4, his RDA is the same as an adult's, even though he grows fast.

If you're concerned that your child's a picky eater and won't get enough nutrients, you may want to give him a vitamin supplement. But be sure to select it carefully, and always make healthy food available to your child. (You never know when he'll start to eat broccoli or salmon.) Above all, don't panic. Some things that seem like nutritional problems are actually normal changes. For example, during a child's second year, his growth rate slows. At about age 10 months, his appetite decreases and stays low into the second year. At this stage, your child may appear thinner and more muscular. In the second and third years, the typical child's belly sticks out and you may notice a slight sway back when he stands.

In the preschool period, the child continues to grow and gain weight. By his fourth year, he usually becomes leaner, losing his belly and slight sway back.

Because a school-age child uses lots of energy, his appetite and food intake increase as he grows. He may become less of a picky eater, although feeding problems may result if you permit activities that interfere with mealtimes, show an overconcern with table manners, or don't give him foods that he likes.

Better than cookies and chips

Lots of children look forward to snacks. But snacks like soda, cookies, and chips can offer too many calories and too few nutrients. If you give your child healthy snacks, you not only help him get all of his nutrients, but you also help him develop good eating habits. Here are some snack suggestions for giving your child more than "empty" calories:

- *peanut butter spread on quarters of a cored, raw apple*
- *banana milkshake (whole milk, banana, and a dab of honey whipped up in a blender)*
- *trail mix. Try a commercial brand or make your own mixture of unsalted peanuts, raisins, sunflower seeds, etc.*
- *unsalted mixed nuts served with fruit juice*
- *frozen yogurt or juice pops. To make your own, pour fruit juice or well-mixed, fruited yogurt in an ice cube tray. When the mix freezes slightly, add a popsicle stick to each cube*
- *carrot and celery sticks with a cottage cheese- or yogurt-based dip.*

If you use your imagination, you'll think of lots more healthy snacks. However, when you shop for snacks, watch out for "junk foods" that masquerade as "health foods." For instance, a chocolate-dipped granola bar may have more calories and more fat per ounce than a chocolate-coated candy bar. So be sure to read the labels on commercial snacks before you buy them.

Special needs of adolescents

A quick, nutritious breakfast

If you don't have time to eat a full-course breakfast, this power-packed drink can give you most of the nutrients and energy you need to start your day right.

Breakfast shake

- *1 cup of milk*
- *1 egg*
- *1 teaspoon vegetable oil*
- *1 to 2 tablespoons wheat germ*
- *1 teaspoon to 2 tablespoons brewer's yeast*
- *2 tablespoons frozen orange juice (or other fruit juice) concentrate*
- *2 tablespoons powdered milk, optional*

Blend ingredients and drink.

More calories and nutrients are required during adolescence than at any other time except infancy. Teenagers experience a growth spurt from about age 12 to 19 for boys and about age 10 to 15 for girls.

Boys add muscle and bone, ending up with about 8% body fat. They need about 2,800 calories daily. Girls add more fat—ending up with about 20% body fat—so they need fewer calories, about 2,200 daily.

Vitamin and mineral shortages

Teenagers with poor eating habits—skipped breakfasts, junk food snacks, irregular meals, fast food meals, and crash diets—can suffer deficiencies in calcium and iron and in Vitamins A, C, B_1, and folic acid.

Calcium requirements are high—1,200 mg daily. Four 8-ounce servings of milk or yogurt can meet this need. But calcium deficiency commonly results when teenagers substitute soft drinks for milk.

Iron deficiency is also a problem. Teenagers require extra iron during growth periods, and girls need to replace iron lost during menstruation. Teenagers should consume 18 mg of iron dily. (See Vitamins and minerals: their function and food sources, pages 30-41.)

To prevent Vitamin C and various Vitamin B deficiencies, teenagers need whole grain breads and

Facts about fast food

Fast foods are almost a staple in many teenagers' diets. But how do they rate nutritionally? Just look. A typical fast food meal, such as a hamburger, French fries, and a shake, supplies adequate protein and some needed vitamins and minerals. However, for the amount of nutrition, fast food meals are high in calories, fat, and sodium, while they're low in fiber, Vitamin A, Vitamin C, and several B vitamins.

To find out exactly what nutrients fast foods contain, review this chart. (Remember: similar items from different chains are comparable.)

	Brand
Apple pie	McDonald's
Burrito, combination	Taco Bell
Chicken, fried drumstick	Kentucky Fried
Chicken, fried wing	Kentucky Fried
Chocolate sundae, med.	Dairy Queen
Dairy Queen cone, med.	Dairy Queen
Filet-o-Fish	McDonald's
Hamburger	McDonald's
Hot dog	Burger King
Onion rings (Brazier)	Dairy Queen
Taco	Taco Bell
Vanilla shake	McDonald's
Whopper	Burger King

cereals, vegetables, and citrus fruit or juice.

Dieting: never too thin

Teenagers, especially girls, fear being overweight. Typically, after a few days on a crash diet, the dieter gorges on potato chips, ice cream, and other high-calorie foods. The crash diet is the problem: avoid it. Instead, develop the habit of eating nutritious foods like skim milk, lean meat, and salads.

Extremes in dieting can do serious harm, as seen in adolescents who develop anorexia nervosa. It's characterized by dedicated dieting, extreme weight loss, and a belief that one is fat. This disorder sometimes occurs with bulimia—obsessive binge eating followed by vomiting (often induced by ipecac syrup, which can eventually poison the dieter) and purging, usually with laxatives.

Needs of athletes

Most athletes need only a well-balanced diet for adequate nutrition. Except for those with nutritional deficiencies, supplements aren't necessary and don't improve athletic performance. Athletes *do* need more potassium, magnesium, and Vitamin B_1, but usually get them by eating more. To replace lost sweat, they should drink water and use more table salt.

Weight (g)	Food energy (K cal)	Protein (g)	Fat (g)	Carbohydrate (g)	Calcium (mg)	Iron (mg)	Potassium (mg)	Sodium (mg)	Vitamin A (IU)	Thiamine (mg)	Riboflavin (mg)	Niacin (mg)	Vitamin C (mg)
91	300	2	19	31	12	0.6	39	414	<69	0.02	0.03	1.3	3
175	404	21	16	43	91	3.7	278	300	1,666	0.34	0.31	4.6	15
54	136	14	8	2	20	0.9	*	†	30	0.04	0.12	2.7	0
45	151	11	10	4	*	0.6	*	†	*	0.03	0.07	*	0
184	300	6	7	53	200	1.1	*	†	300	0.06	0.26	0	0
142	230	6	7	35	200	0	*	†	300	0.09	0.26	0	0
131	402	15	23	34	105	1.8	293	709	152	0.28	0.28	3.9	4
99	257	13	9	30	63	3	234	526	231	0.23	0.23	5.1	2
*	291	11	17	23	40	2	170	841	0	0.04	0.02	2	0
85	300	6	17	33	20	0.4	16	†	0	0.09	0	0.4	2
83	186	15	8	14	120	2.5	143	79	120	0.09	0.16	2.9	0
289	323	10	8	52	346	0.2	499	250	346	0.12	0.66	0.6	<3
*	606	29	32	32	37	6	653	909	641	0.02	0.03	5.2	13

* Data unavailable   † Content varies   < less than

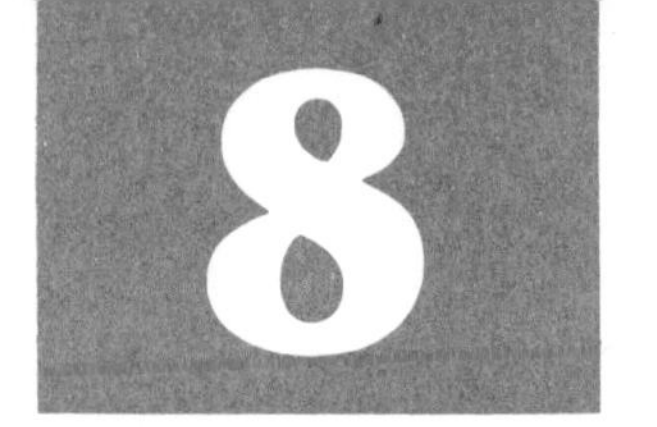

Diet programs

Your calorie needs

Simply, a calorie is a unit of measure. It describes the amount of heat or energy a certain food will produce when your body uses it.

The list below shows the calories people need to maintain their body weight. As you'll see, young adults need more energy—and more calories—because they're more active. Older adults' energy needs decrease as their activity levels decrease and their metabolism slows.

	AGE	CALORIE NEEDS
Men (average: 154 lb [69.3 kg]; 70″ [177.8 cm])	19 to 22	2,500-3,000
	23 to 50	2,300-3,100
	51 to 75	2,000-2,800
	over 75	1,650-2,450
Women* (average: 20 lb. [54 kg]; 64″ [162.6 cm])	19 to 22	1,700-2,500
	23 to 50	1,600-2,400
	51 to 75	1,400-2,200
	over 75	1,200-2,000

*Pregnant women need 300 more calories a day; and breast-feeding women need 500 extra calories a day.

For most people, the best diet is getting a certain number of helpings from the four basic food groups: milk, meat, fruit-vegetable, and bread-cereal. Within those basic boundaries, if you choose wisely, you should be able to meet most, if not all, of your daily dietary nutritional needs. But some people, for a variety of reasons, can't or won't eat a good, basic diet. The three most common reasons for deviating from that diet are a desire to lose weight, restrictions imposed by personal beliefs, and restrictions imposed for medical reasons. Of these, the most common in America today is the desire to lose weight.

Now, excess weight should concern all of us because it is a contributing factor in heart disease and other ailments. Perhaps, however, it has become a little too much of a concern (excessive thinness isn't healthy either) and for the wrong reasons. Most people tend to diet to look better, not necessarily to get healthier, and they often don't recognize the pitfalls that weight-loss dieting can create for health.

Counting calories

Most weight-loss programs simply reduce the number of calories you take in each day. Yet caloric need can vary from person to person. A six-foot-four linebacker might be dieting if he cut his intake back to under 3,000 calories a day, while a jockey in training might want to keep his intake under 1,500. Usually, a weight-loss diet is 1,200 calories or fewer a day. Anything below 700 or 800 calories a day is essentially a starvation diet and

The problems with diets

When you change your diet, you alter the amount of nutrients coming into your body. Below is a list of the major common diets and what vitamins and minerals they can lead you to be low in. On these diets, you'll have to plan your meals carefully.

Diet	***Possible deficiency***
Low calorie (below 1,200)	*All vitamins and minerals*
Low carbohydrates	*All vitamins and minerals*
Low protein	*Pantothenate*
High protein	*Calcium*
Low sodium	*Pantothenate*
Low sugar	*Riboflavin*
Low cholesterol	*Vitamins A, D, and E*
Strict vegetarian	*Iron, Vitamin B_{12}*

Variety is the spice

Some enthusiastic dieters eat nothing but a can of tuna and part of a head of lettuce for dinner every night in their effort to lose weight. While they might lose a few pounds this way, they're also going to be losing ground nutritionally. Every diet, whether it's just calorie counting or a complex program of high or low proteins and carbohydrates, should always have variety, following the basic food groups. Not only will this ensure greater nutritional balance, it'll also make the diet less boring and probably easier to follow.

can be dangerous. But even at better than subsistence levels, dieting can undermine your health.

In Chapter 5 we saw how the elderly, simply because they eat less, get fewer vitamins and minerals. This is true of dieters, too. At 1,200 or fewer calories daily, you might get enough food to keep you going, but for good health you would still need your regular numbers of vitamins and minerals. For this reason, if you plan to lower your intake to any significant degree (a change of more than 500 calories—we all tend to go up and down a bit normally), you really should pay attention to eating foods high in vitamins and minerals and low in calories (like broccoli and lean white chicken meat), and you might also want to take a basic multivitamin and multimineral preparation.

Weight-loss dieting isn't just a matter of eating less. If it were, then all those diet books wouldn't have been selling so many millions of copies these past few years. Three popular forms of diet are high protein/low carbohydrate, low protein/high carbohydrate, and high protein complex carbohydrate. All have their own theories on how weight can be lost (for example, high protein/low carbohydrate diets aim to deprive your body of all forms of sugar, even starches, so that it starts to burn fat), and all have their strong and vocal supporters. One thing—regardless of whether they're high this or high that, these diets are low in calories, and as such, all are deficient in some vitamins and minerals. The problem is simple: when you eat less food, you get fewer nutrients. Unless you're a good planner, you'll deprive yourself of essential vitamins and minerals as you diet.

If you embark on one of these plans, you can safeguard yourself with a multivitamin and multimineral every day, with perhaps some extra Vitamin C if your diet doesn't allow you many fruits or vegetables, and maybe some extra calcium and Vitamin D if you're not allowed milk or cheese.

(continued on page 76)

Determining your body frame

Before you start on a weight loss diet, determine your type of body frame. Why? Because you'll need this information to find out how much you should weigh. Use the graph to compare your wrist measurement with your height. This comparison reveals your body frame type.

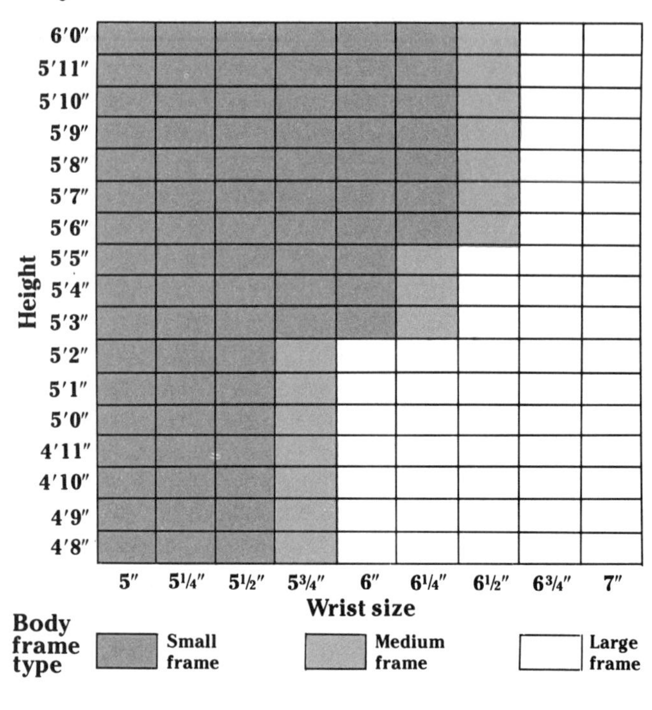

Your ideal body weight

Because fitness is related to weight, you'll want to compare your weight with the range for your age, height, and sex. If you're seriously over or under the average weight reading, you may have a medical problem and should consult a doctor, especially if you're considering a fitness program.

Men				Women			
Height	Small build (±4%)	Medium build (±5%)	Large build (±6%)	Height	Small build (±4%)	Medium build (±5%)	Large build (±6%)
5'2"	123	131	138	4'9"	107	114	122
3"	127	135	143	10"	109	116	124
4"	131	139	147	11"	111	118	126
5"	134	142	151	5'0"	114	121	129
6"	138	146	155	1"	117	124	132
7"	141	150	159	2"	120	128	136
8"	145	154	163	3"	123	131	139
9"	149	158	168	4"	127	135	144
10"	154	162	172	5"	131	139	148
11"	158	167	177	6"	134	142	151
6'0"	163	172	182	7"	138	146	155
1"	169	177	187	8"	141	150	159
2"	174	182	192	9"	145	153	162

*10 top low-calorie, high-nutrient foods**

Food and portion size	*Nutrients provided*
Asparagus, 4 fresh spears	Vitamins A, B_1, B_2, B_6, and C; folic acid; magnesium; potassium
Broccoli, ½ cup fresh	Vitamins A, B_1, B_2, B_6, and C; folic acid; calcium; phosphorus; magnesium; iron; zinc; potassium
Brussels sprouts, ½ cup fresh	Vitamins B_2, B_6, and C; niacin; folic acid; phosphorus; magnesium; iron; potassium
Cantaloupe, ¼ melon	Vitamins A, B_1, B_2, B_6, and C; niacin; phosphorus; magnesium; iron; sodium; potassium
Clams, 3 ounces canned	Vitamins B_1, B_2, B_6, B_{12}, and C; niacin; calcium; phosphorus; iron; zinc; sodium; potassium
Pepper, 1 medium	Vitamins A, B_6, and C; magnesium; iron; phosphorus
Sauerkraut, ½ cup	Vitamins B_6 and C; calcium; iron; sodium; potassium
Spinach, ½ cup cooked	Vitamins A, B_2, B_6, and C; folic acid; calcium; magnesium; iron; potassium
Tomato, 1 fresh medium	Vitamins A, B_1, and C; niacin; magnesium; iron; potassium
Wheat germ, 1 tablespoon	Vitamins B_1 and B_6; folic acid; phosphorus; magnesium; iron; zinc

**45 calories or less per serving*

Vegetarians

The most common diet around the world is followed by those who believe that eating meat is wrong or by those who think it's healthier for them not to eat meat. But there are certain things that meat and animal products give use that plants can't, such as complete protein.

Strict vegetarians will also lack Vitamin B_{12} in their diets, because it can only be found in animal products. Iron, although found in both plants and animals, is far more effective when animal in origin. Fortunately, most vegetarians are well aware that they have special nutritional needs and make sure that these needs are met by taking supplements or, in the case of iron, eating extra spinach.

Special diets

The last main form of diet is the kind dictated by medical needs. When on a low-cholesterol diet, you should be aware that Vitamin A and the other fat-soluble vitamins are found in the fatty portions of food. So, if you're no longer eating liver because of its cholesterol content, make sure you're making up for it with a few extra carrots and some broccoli. Cutting back on your salt with a low-sodium diet may help lower your blood pressure. But it can also boost your need for pantothenate, as can low-protein diets, which stress your adrenal system. People on diets to control ulcers or diabetes should know that they might be low in riboflavin. People allergic to certain foods will have to eat other foods high in the nutrients they're missing. All of these losses can be covered by eating more of certain vitamin-rich foods, or by taking supplements.

You generally get your nutrition through what you eat; so, when you change what you eat, how much you eat, or both, you have to make sure that you're meeting your daily nutritional needs.

How vegetarians can get essential amino acids

Essential Amino Acids
Grains
Barley, pearl
Bread, whole wheat
Corn meal
Corn-soy grits
Macaroni or spaghetti
Millet
Oatmeal
Rice
Tortillas
Wheat bran
Wheat germ
Legumes
Beans: navy, red, etc.
Chickpeas
Lentils
Lima beans
Lupine
Split peas
Soybeans
Nuts and seeds
Almonds
Cashews
Coconut
Peanuts
Sesame meal
Sunflower seeds

Fad diets and your health

Certain fad diets are not only low in vitamins and minerals; they may also cause serious side effects.

The liquid protein diet has actually caused death. No one should use it with-

Animal products usually contain complete protein with all eight essential amino acids. Except for soybeans, the strict vegetarian (or *vegan*) diet includes few foods that by themselves offer complete protein. To get it, vegetarians must combine foods until they get all 8 essential amino acids in one meal. (For example, red beans and rice for corn meal bread with split pea soup.) This chart shows which ones exist in different foods.

Isoleucine	Leucine	Lysine	Methionine	Phenylalanine	Threonine	Tryptophan	Valine
■	■		■	■		■	■
■	■		■	■	■	■	■
■	■		■	■	■		■
■	■		■	■	■	■	■
■	■		■	■		■	■
■	■		■	■	■	■	■
■	■		■	■	■	■	■
■	■		■	■	■	■	■
■	■				■		■
■	■		■	■		■	■
■	■	■		■	■	■	■
■	■	■		■	■	■	■
■	■	■		■	■		■
■	■	■		■	■	■	■
■	■	■		■	■	■	■
	■				■		■
■	■	■		■	■	■	■
■	■	■	■	■	■	■	■
■	■		■	■		■	■
■	■		■	■	■	■	■
■	■		■	■	■	■	■
■	■			■		■	■
■	■		■	■		■	
■	■		■	■	■	■	■

out medical supervision. Misuse can result in muscle breakdown, fatigue, diarrhea or constipation, dizziness, fainting, muscle cramps, nausea, dry skin, low blood sugar, and changes in heart rhythm.

In the final stage of the Zen macrobiotic diet (when only rice is eaten), side effects can include Vitamin C deficiency, protein deficiency, calcium deficiency, emaciation, loss of kidney function, anemia, fatigue, low resistance to infection, and heavy vaginal discharge—among others.

When you eliminate all carbohydrates, as in the low carbohydrate diet, ketosis occurs. This condition increases the body's use of its fat stores and stresses the liver and kidneys. The diet can also cause kidney or bladder stones, and high cholesterol levels.

9 Exercise

One big benefit
Heavy exercisers are about the only adults who may have the luxury of being able to eat extra sugars and starches without fear of gaining weight.

Along with watching what you eat, exercising is about the best thing you can do for yourself. But if you just exercise, without watching what you eat, you're only doing yourself about half as much good. For one thing, exercise puts certain demands on your body that you have to compensate for.

One of them is calories. The more you exercise, whether it be a four-mile run, an hour-long aerobics class, or a regular game of racquetball, the more calories your body's going to burn. Up to a point that can be good, especially if you want to lose weight (it works better than dieting). But if you want to exercise a lot and not lose weight, you're going to have to eat more, too. People who engage in this kind of workout need more calories and, especially, more protein and carbohydrates (which is why runners often "carbo load"—eat a lot of carbohydrates—over the days leading up to a marathon). Other demands increase as well.

Water-soluble vitamins are the first to be affected by exercise because your body will flush them out with your sweat. Vitamins B_{12} and C are particularly susceptible to being lost through your pores during exercise, as are riboflavin and thiamine.

Heat can accelerate the loss of these vitamins. Contrary to popular belief, though, you don't lose that much sodium through sweating when you exercise in the heat, so there's no need to take salt pills (you'd only get such a sodium deficiency in severe heat with severe dehydration, and if it's that hot out—high 80s or above—and the humidity is high, you shouldn't be exercising at all). However, you can lose potassium and magnesium, which keep your muscles working properly.

Another mineral that may have something to do with how well your muscles work is iron.

Certain exercise regimens demand certain diets. One of the most common is a high-protein diet, used by weight lifters and body builders (although many question whether or not this does them any good). This diet can result in low levels of calcium, which must be replaced.

When it's hot

When it's too hot—high 80s or above—and the humidity is high, don't exercise outdoors. If you really want to burn off some calories, turn on an air conditioner and do some aerobics and stretching. Or, if you're near a pool, lake, or ocean, swimming is a cool alternative to running around in the hot sun. Exercising even in moderate heat—70s and above—can pose problems, the chief of which is dehydration, so make sure you get plenty of water. Also make sure you're stoked up on Vitamin C and potassium, as they wash out with your sweat quite rapidly. Don't worry about taking salt tablets—you'd only lose a big amount of sodium if you were to exercise strenuously in severe heat for an extended period of time, something you shouldn't do in the first place. You might want to eat an orange or a banana: they'll replace your potassium and give you an energy boost.

People who exercise may need a basic multivitamin and multimineral. Heavy exercisers, as much as or more than any group, must be concerned about getting a balanced diet because the demands they place on their bodies are greater.

Why exercise?

Some benefits of a regular exercise program are obvious: improved appearance, weight control, and overall better health. But others are more hidden—for example, physical exercise throughout life can actually slow the loss of calcium from the body and help prevent bone degeneration, or *osteoporosis*, in old age. Regular exercise can not only extend your life—middle-aged people with desk jobs who don't exercise are twice as susceptible to heart attacks as those who do—but can also improve the quality of your life.

Your exercise program

A good exercise routine contracts and stretches all your body's major muscle groups, improving your strength and flexibility, and raises your heart rate, making your heart and lungs stronger and more resilient and improving your stamina and overall fitness level. For your exercise routine to be effective, you need to perform it at least three times a week, a minimum of 20 continuous minutes each session, during which you maintain your heartbeat (pulse) between 70 and 85 percent of its maximum capability. To help you stick to your routine, choose exercises that you enjoy.

Aerobic training level

For best effects in aerobic exercise, you must work a little harder than what is comfortable for you, but a lot less than all-out exertion. During exercise, use your watch to count the number of pulse beats in a 10-second interval. Then refer to the chart below. Find your age in the left column. Read across to find your 70 percent and 85 percent of maximum pulse rates during a 10-second reading.

For the most beneficial results, maintain your pulse during exercise between the 70 and 85 percent figures.

If you want to know what your 1-minute pulse rate should be, multiply your 10-second count by 6.

Ten-second pulse rate after exercise

Age	70 percent	85 percent
20	23	28
25	23	28
30	22	27
35	22	26
40	21	26
45	20	25
50	20	24
55	19	23
60	19	23
65	18	22
70	18	21

Benefits of 20-minute activities

This chart shows common activities, the calories they burn, and their value in improving stamina, flexibility, and strength.

Activity	Calories	Stamina*	Flexibility	Strength
Easy walking	60	M	M	M
Light housework	90	M	F	F
Light gardening (weeding, etc.)	90	M	F	F
Golf (flat course)	90	M	F	M
Brisk walking	100	F	F	F
Badminton	115	F	G	F
Horseback riding	115	F	G	F
Gymnastics	140	F	E	F
Heavy gardening (digging, etc.)	140	F	G	E
Dancing	160	F	G	M
Easy jogging	160	F	F	F
Tennis	160	G	G	F
Ice skating	160	G	G	F
Skiing (downhill)	160	G	G	F
Skiing (cross-country)	180	E	G	G
Rowing	180	E	G	G
Soccer	180	G	G	G
Football	180	G	F	G
Racquetball or handball	200	G	G	F
Brisk jogging	210	E	F	G
Bicycling	220	E	F	G
Swimming	240	E	E	E

KEY: E = excellent, G = good, F = fair, M = minimal

* *Excellent ratings occur when pulse is maintained between 70 and 85% of maximum.*

Determining your fitness level

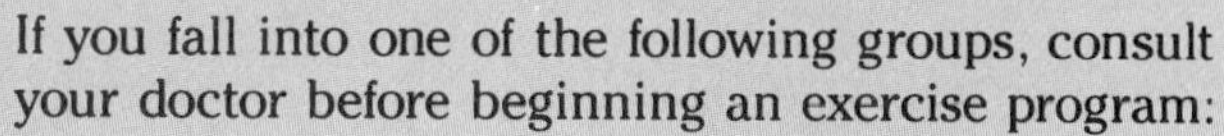

If you fall into one of the following groups, consult your doctor before beginning an exercise program:
- those over age 45 who haven't exercised regularly since early adulthood, or people over age 60
- heavy smokers
- obese persons
- people with a chronic health problem such as diabetes, hypertension, or heart, lung, or kidney disease
- people who rate "unfit" or "poor" on the step test.

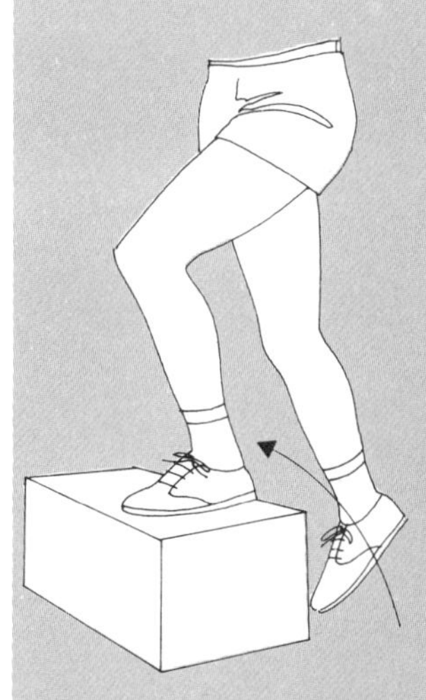

One quick way to determine your overall fitness level is the step test.

Begin the test by walking steadily up three flights of stairs of 15 to 20 steps each. If you have to pause to catch your breath, or if you're so breathless when you reach the top that you can't talk normally, you are unfit. Don't attempt the next part of the test, and see your doctor before starting any exercise program.

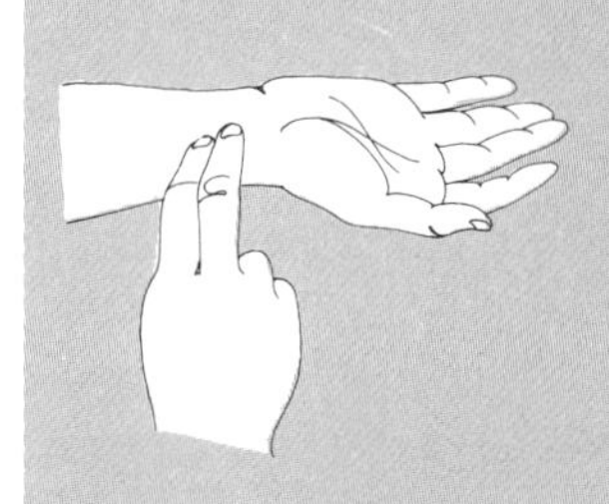

If you pass the first part of the test, move on to the second part. Stand on the floor level facing the stairs. Step up on the bottom step with one foot, bring up the other foot, then step back down to the floor. Repeat at a rate of 24 times a minute for 3 minutes. (Caution: if you start to feel dizzy, faint, or nauseated, stop the test immediately.) Stop after 3 minutes, wait exactly 1 minute, then count your pulse for the next 15 seconds. Use the chart below to determine your fitness rating.

Fitness ratings for men and women

15-second pulse count				Fitness rating
Women under age 45	***Women over age 45***	***Men under age 45***	***Men over age 45***	
below 20	below 21	below 18	below 19	*excellent*
20-22	21-23	18-20	19-21	*good*
23-28	24-29	21-25	22-26	*average*
above 28	above 29	above 25	above 26	*poor*

10 Modern life

The low-down on alcohol

Many people drink alcohol for its relaxing or stimulating effects, and some studies assert that 1 to 2 drinks a day can decrease your risk of heart disease. But are these potential benefits worth the known risks? Not if you find that you're increasing the amount you drink. Excessive, long-term alcohol use can:

- *deplete the body of vital vitamins and minerals*
- *cause organ damage*
- *hamper the liver's ability to process fat*
- *destroy brain cells*
- *cause veins to rupture.*

Vitamins and minerals, those relatively new discoveries, may help us cope with some of the hazards of modern life. For example, vitamins and minerals may help us deal with stress. Pantothenate, in particular, has been shown to greatly improve how rats cope in stressful situations—and it may help you contend with your own "rat race." Vitamin A and Vitamin C, along with calcium, may also help us diffuse tension and relax a little bit better.

Vitamin muggers

While some things in modern life, like stress, simply demand more of us, other things actually steal vitamins and minerals from us. One of the biggest nutritional muggers is smoking, which is not only linked to heart disease and cancer, but also robs us of Vitamin C (reports indicate that this may be what makes it so carcinogenic, because C effectively blocks certain cancer-causing substances like nitrosamines). As the US Surgeon-Generals have been saying for years, smoking is hazardous to your health, and if you do smoke, you really should try to stop. If you can't, then make sure you're taking enough extra Vitamin C to make up for the amount cigarettes take from you.

The biggest mugger of vitamins and minerals is alcohol. Whether in beer, wine, or liquor, alcohol is a toxic substance (which is why, when we drink it, we can get "intoxicated"). As such, your liver works overtime to detoxify it—which is why prolonged abuse of alcohol can damage your liver. In this effort, your body is drained of five key B-complex vitamins—thiamine, riboflavin, B_6, B_{12} and folic acid—as well as magnesium and zinc. So, if you are a regular drinker, you might be wise to take some extra B-complex vitamins as well as magnesium and zinc.

Two other popular drinks are also notorious vitamin and minerals muggers—coffee and tea. The caffeine in both of them destroys thiamine, and too much tea can lower the amount of iron your body can absorb and use.

Avoiding these vitamin muggers isn't difficult—none of them is essential to you. Food, however, is essential,

Surprising sources of caffeine

You know that coffee and tera contain large amounts of caffeine. But did you know about these other sources? Cocoa, chocolate, and many soft drinks (both colas and non-colas) are high in caffeine. And, perhaps most surprisingly, normal doses of many over-the-counter drugs—notably pain relievers, such as Anacin, Midol, and Excedrin, and diet pills, such as Dexatrim—may contain more caffeine than a cup of coffee.

and, unfortunately, it's in food that one of the biggest nutritional hazards of modern life can be found.

Modern food

Americans ate differently 100 years ago. While you couldn't get tomatoes year-round like we can now, the fruits and vegetables you did get were fresh, local, and mostly free of preservatives. And most grains weren't processed nearly as much. And so, along with more processing and greater convenience has come a decline in the vitamin and mineral content in our food.

With refrigeration and long-distance transportation of food, people *could* eat better now than ever before. What's disturbing is that in the quest for ease, we opt for what's fast, not what's best. The fast foods that the major chains churn out are by no means totally devoid of nutritional value. It's just that if you consume one-third of your daily caloric intake in the form of mass-produced hamburgers with french fries, you get just a fraction of the nutritional value you would by preparing yourself a hamburger at home, served on whole grain bread, with a baked potato and a salad. You could also then control the amount of salt you eat.

Stress

Stress is just one of the many mental problems that face us in modern life. The B-complex vitamins in particular have been shown to have a very specific connection to how evenly our brains and nervous system operate, and when we're low in the B vitamins, our personalities, how we feel, and how we behave can be affected. Making sure we're getting what we need of the B complex, and maybe a little extra pantothenate, can help us cool off and even out some of the more jarring bumps and slumps of modern living. The slumps also may have something to do with the depression that accompanies iron deficiency anemia, a hazard that women in particular should be on the lookout for.

Freedom from stress has an important impact on overall health, because stress seems to weaken the immune system and lower our resistance to illness. For a rough idea of how stress has affected your life during the past year, take a look at Evaluating stress on page 84.

A simple plan for better health

There are three keys to getting healthy and staying that way—diet, exercise, and adequate vitamin and mineral intake. We have long known that the first is important. From the time we were children we've heard

(continued on page 86)

Evaluating stress

To evaluate your stress level, use the scale shown here. This is the Social Readjustment Rating Scale devised in 1967 by Thomas H. Holmes, MD, and Richard H. Rahe, MD. It rates important life changes according to the amount of stress they evoke and how much time a person needs to adjust. To use it, simply go down the list of items and circle those events that have happened to you in the past year. Then add up your score. Check this chart to find out—roughly—your chances of developing a major illness in the next 2 years.

150 or below	*1 chance in 3*
150-300	*1 chance in 2*
300+	*90% chance*

Event	***Rating***
Death of spouse	100 ______
Divorce	73 ______
Marital separation	65 ______
Jail term	63 ______
Death of close family member	63 ______
Personal injury or illness	53 ______
Marriage	50 ______
Fired from work	47 ______
Marital reconciliation	45 ______
Retirement	45 ______
Change in health of family member	44 ______
Pregnancy	40 ______
Sex difficulties	39 ______
Gain of new family member	39 ______
Business readjustment	39 ______
Change in financial state	38 ______
Death of close friend	37 ______
Change to different line of work	36 ______
Change in number of arguments with spouse	35 ______
New mortgage	31 ______
Foreclosure of mortgage or loan	30 ______
Change in responsibilities at work	29 ______
Son or daughter leaving home	29 ______
Trouble with in-laws	29 ______
Outstanding personal achievement	28 ______
Spouse begins or stops work	26 ______
Begin or end school	26 ______
Change in living conditions	25 ______
Revision of personal habits	24 ______
Trouble with boss	23 ______
Change in work hours or conditions	20 ______
Change in residence	20 ______
Change in schools	20 ______
Change in recreation	19 ______
Change in religious commitment	19 ______
Change in social activities	18 ______
Small mortgage or loan	17 ______
Change in sleeping habits	16 ______
Change in number of family get-togethers	15 ______
Change in eating habits	15 ______
Vacation	12 ______
Christmas/Hanukkah/New Year's	12 ______
Minor violations of the law	11 ______
	Total: ______

Relieving stress

When stress builds, you may find exercising is a good way to relax. The exercises shown here are simple to perform and won't take much time to do. They'll help relieve tension in your neck and back—common trouble spots. Do these exercises gently and slowly. Stop if they cause pain.

Back roll. Sit in a chair, feet about a foot apart. Slowly roll forward from your waist so that your face rests between your knees and your arms hang toward the floor, then slowly roll back up, feeling each vertebra as it rolls back up against the chair. Sit tall, stretch up, and then roll forward again and repeat. This is an exercise that you can do several times a day, even while sitting at your desk.

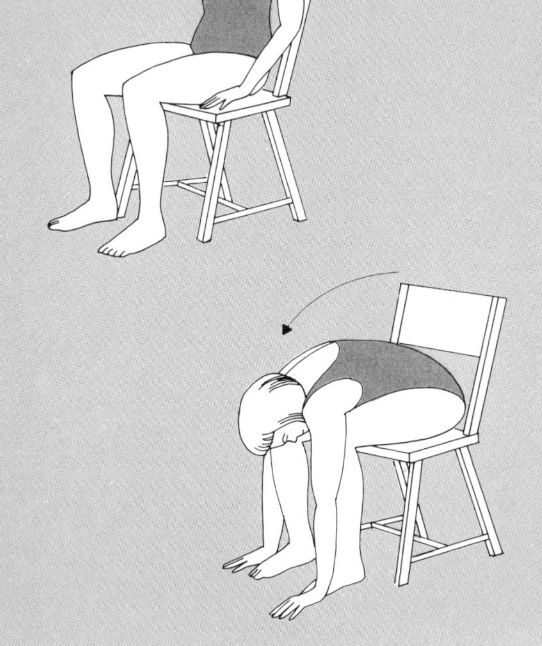

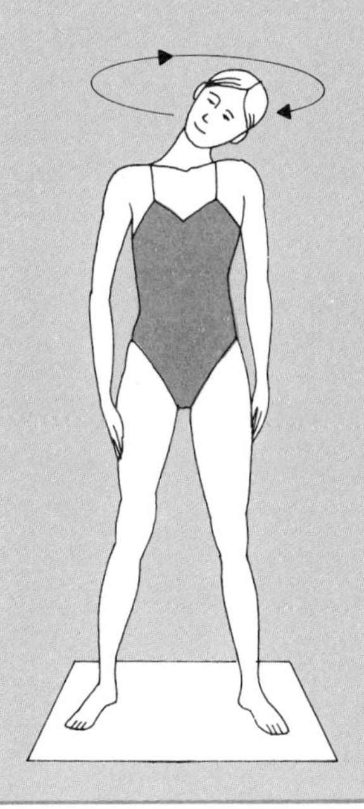

Neck roll. Standing upright, feet apart, *slowly* roll you head from one side to the other. Do 3 rolls in each direction. You can also do this exercise while sitting in a chair.

Junk food

There's good news and bad news about junk food like potato chips, soft drinks, and their ilk. The good news is that with the increased health consciousness of the past few years, manufacturers have tried to create better *junk foods. At the supermarket you'll now see potato chips with no salt or preservatives, perhaps prepared with less oil than their predecessors. And you'll see soft drinks with no sugar, no caffeine, and occasionally no sodium.*

The bad news is that until manufacturers coat their potato chips with vitamins and minerals and dump more of the same into their soft drinks, junk foods will remain junk—providing little or no nutrition.

Processing leeches foods of their nutrients, and junk foods are about the most processed foods you can find. If you look at the nutritional information on a bag of potato chips, you'll see that you'd have to eat about a crate of them to gain any nutritional value. What junk food provides are "empty calories"—lots of sugar and carbohydrates, but few nutrients. By all means, if you're in the middle of the desert and all you have to survive on is a bag of cheese snacks and a bottle of root beer, go ahead. But, in this land of plenty, satisfy yourself with other nutritious snack foods like nuts, fresh popcorn, and raisins and other dried fruits.

"you are what you eat" and have been exhorted to eat a balanced diet of foods that are "good for us." But even more attention has been paid to diet recently, and we've found that what was once common sense has a wealth of scientific data behind it.

Tailoring your diet

What *your* diet should be depends on *your* needs. If you're an athlete you might want to eat more protein and carbohydrates than the next guy; if you're a breast-feeding mother you'll want more cheese and milk; if you have high blood pressure you'll want to restrict the amount of salt in the foods you eat. Even with all these variations, the old standard of taking roughly twice as much each day from the fruit-vegetable and bread-cereal groups as you do from the milk and meat groups still applies. It's your choice within these groups that is so very important. You choose foods, not just for their vitamin and mineral contents but also for their protein, calories, carbohydrates, taste, and personal appeal. For example, while liver, in terms of vitamins and minerals, is about *the* best thing for you to eat, it also has a lot of calories, is very high in cholesterol, and has a distinctive taste and texture.

Tailoring your diet around your vitamin and mineral needs doesn't mean all of a sudden you have to go out and start eating weird things like yeast or lecithin. Nor does it mean you have to start eating foods you don't like. Choose the foods you like, but do so according to what they contain. Just because you don't like liver or spinach doesn't mean you can't get your Vitamin A or iron. Just look down the lists beginning on page 30. For Vitamin A you can also go to carrots, broccoli, cantaloupe, even watermelon. Iron is abundant in ground beef, turkey, and peas.

Processing and preparation are the two big foes of

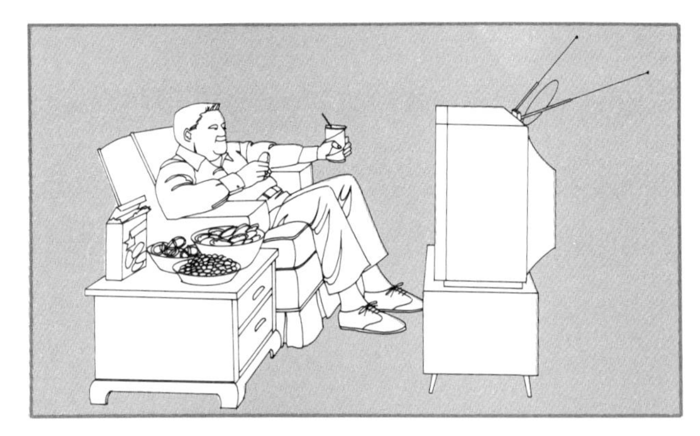

No shortcuts

You won't find any shortcuts to good health. Just as vitamin supplements are no substitute for a balanced diet, fancy "exercise" machines or "miracle reducers" can't compete with good old-fashioned exercise. You can't get fit by lying on a table that shakes, wearing a belt that vibrates, or zipping yourself into a plastic suit that "melts the pounds away." You don't have to run out and enter a triathlon, but you do need vigorous, sustained physical exertion to improve and maintain your fitness level.

vitamins and minerals in your food. The small amount of extra time it takes for you to prepare your own meal from fresh ingredients, instead of using canned or frozen foods, will bring you astoundingly greater benefit. And when you do prepare your own food, wash fruits and vegetables but avoid soaking them (water can leech out some vitamins), eat most of your fruits raw (many vegetables can be eaten raw too), and steam (but not for too long), stir fry, or bake the others.

Planning your exercise program

What your body needs most after good food is good exercise. The average person should get at least 20 minutes of fairly strenuous exercise, at least three or more times a week. The cardinal rule of all exercise is to start slow—and don't be discouraged. If you start walking a few miles every other day, you'll be amazed at what you'll be able to do in a few months. And set yourself reasonable goals. Accomplishing them will make you feel better mentally as well as physically.

Getting your vitamins and minerals

The most neglected part of a simple fitness plan is careful attention to vitamins and minerals. Isn't it best to meet all your nutritional needs through what you eat, rather than swallowing a tablet? The answer, unequivocally, is *yes*. Vitamins and minerals in food come with other things, like proteins, carbohydrates, and fiber, that are also very good for you. Still, unless you're very careful about your diet, the way you live may increase your vitamin and mineral needs beyond what you're getting from your diet. You may need a vitamin and mineral supplement.

There's a lot more to be learned about vitamins and minerals. Not only do we not know everything they can do for us, but we're also not sure if we've discovered all the vitamins and minerals that are important to our health. There are tantalizing possibilities that vitamins and minerals may play key roles in preventing cancer, controlling heart disease, helping us heal, keeping us illness-free, clearing up skin, and a host of other problems. But vitamins and minerals aren't a panacea. They can't do everything. Where we live, the work we do, and the traits we've inherited are all factors that have just as much of an impact on our health as what we eat does. But remember: a simple three-part plan of watching what you eat, exercising, and tending to your vitamin and mineral needs is the easiest way to get healthy and stay that way.

11

What vitamins and minerals can't do

Vitamins and minerals: A miracle cure?

Some enthusiasts would have you believe that vitamins and minerals can cure everything from cancer to the common cold—that vitamins and minerals can work a kind of "miracle cure." Unfortunately, that's just not so. But vitamins and minerals can *do some fairly remarkable things.*

For instance, taking the right vitamins or minerals can often reverse the effects of a deficiency disease, such as scurvy or beriberi. Although vitamin and mineral deficiencies are rare in countries where nutritious food is abundant, they can occur when people limit their intake in an abnormal way.

Vitamins and minerals can also reduce the risk of disease by keeping up your resistance to infection. They may even help speed recovery when you're sick.

In addition, we know that vitamins and minerals can do great things to help you keep your energy high, keep you healthy, and perhaps make you feel good. That's plenty, without any claims for miracles.

This is the area in which vitamins and minerals have been getting into trouble. When some people start saying that Vitamin C can *cure* cancer, and that Vitamin E can *halt* aging, other people get understandably suspicious. For one thing, such claims are potentially dangerous. Such is the case of the "vitamin" laetrile, an extract of apricot pits. When rumor spread that it could cure cancer, doctors and medical researchers were skeptical; they worried that people would forsake the conventional cancer treatments that have proven to be somewhat effective. (Laetrile hasn't been found to have any effect on cancer whatsoever, and, since it's part cyanide, it *can* poison you.) This worry that people will ignore conventional treatments that work casts a pall over vitamin and mineral claims.

Scientific proof or wishful thinking?

For example, just because thiamine and niacin may have something to do with warding off heart disease doesn't mean that if you're getting those two vitamins you can stop thinking about your heart. The major illnesses discussed here all have two things in common—none of them is caused by *one* factor, and none of them can be prevented or treated by *one* factor. In fact, if vitamins and minerals do play a role, it might be important, even a key one, yet it might be a small part of the whole picture. With heart disease, for example, while you may benefit from high levels of certain vitamins and minerals, you're going to do yourself much greater good if you cut back on fats and sugar, don't smoke, reduce your stress level, and exercise regularly.

Yet some people claim that vitamin and minerals can cure everything from arthritis to senility. For the most part, these claims are more the result of wishful thinking than scientific proof. But our minds shouldn't be shut—some parts of the claims may turn out to be fruitful. The properties of vitamins and minerals are only now being fully explored, and when you consider what we already know about them, and what

What the future may bring

We don't know everything about vitamins and minerals. But we have every reason to expect some important discoveries, as researchers continue to explore the potential uses of vitamins and minerals.

For instance, researchers are investigating the connection between Vitamin C and interferon—a protein that helps keep viruses from penetrating healthy human tissue cells. Vitamin C may play arole in the body's synthesis of interferon and may work with interferon to keep cells healthy.

The role of Vitamin E in treating benign breast cycts also looks promising. In one study, 26 women with fibrocystic breast disease were given 600 I.U. of Vitamin E daily for 8 weeks, with dramatic results. Twelve women showed fair-to-moderate improvement, and in 10 women, cysts disappeared completely or almost completely.

Clearly, more research is in order to reveal the full potential of vitamin and mineral therapy. But with these and other studies currently underway, the future looks bright.

a tremendous effect they can have on our health, we have reason to expect additional important discoveries.

Vitamins and minerals aren't a panacea. They can't cure all ills. There have been many lofty claims, and most of them have been simply wrong. Here are some of the things vitamins and minerals *can't* do:

Vitamin A won't cure acne

Dermatologists are quite interested in what certain vitamins and minerals, particularly zinc, might do for acne sufferers, but despite what you've heard, Vitamin A is not on that list.

Vitamin B_{12} won't give you energy

For a while there was a fad about getting B_{12} shots to perk you up. People who got them said they gave them an energy burst. But the shots were never tested for "placebo effect"—maybe the people felt better just because they *wanted* to feel more energetic. As far as anyone knows, the only people who'll get more energy from a B_{12} injection are people who are clinically deficient in the vitamin to the point of getting the symptoms of pernicious anemia.

Vitamin C won't cure the common cold

By bolstering your immune system, Vitamin C may help keep you from getting a cold in the first place, but once a cold has its talons in you, it's going to have to run its course. However, Vitamin C might help you feel a little better a little faster.

Vitamin E won't stop you from getting old

Someday, perhaps, there may be a cure for the most common of all progressive diseases—aging—but don't count on Vitamin E being part of the cure. Vitamin E has been credited with more healing powers and has been treated with more exaggeration and hyperbole than almost all the other vitamins and minerals combined.

Vitamin E won't improve your sex life

When Vitamin E was completely removed from the diet of rats in a lab, the rats became sterile, and maybe that's how E got its reputation as the "sex vitamin." So far there's no evidence that it will help with endurance, libido, frigidity, or potency.

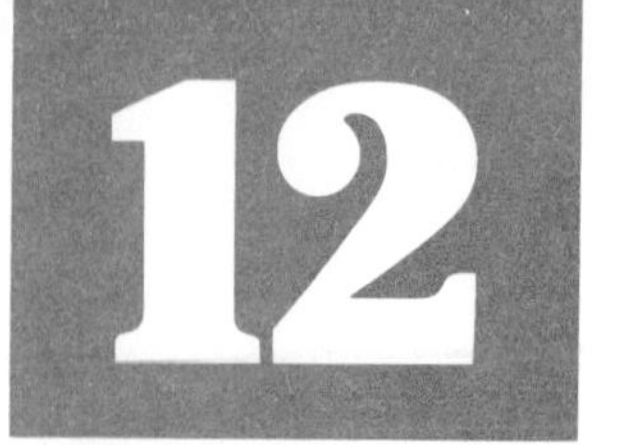

Vitamin and mineral precautions

Megadoses: pros and cons

*A lot of attention has been given to people who claim that large doses (*mega-doses*) of vitamins will cure a variety of ills. Although some therapeutic benefit has been reported, it hasn't been entirely verified. The logic of megadoses is simple: if something is good for you, more of it is better. We know, however, that high doses of fat-soluble vitamins that your body stores can do you harm. There's also evidence that any extra you take of a water-soluble vitamin is just flushed out by your system.*

Assuming that vitamins and minerals are therapeutic, the other argument for megadoses of vitamins and minerals is that they are better for your body than drugs because they're natural and not foreign to your system. On the other hand, there isn't anything "natural" about eating 4,000 mg. of Vitamin C every day.

If you're thinking about taking megadoses of vitamins as a cure, remember that their value is really more curative (about all they cure is their own deficiencies). With all these questions, anyone considering embarking on a megadose program really should consult a doctor first.

Vitamins and minerals aren't dangerous, but you'll want to follow two basic rules for vitamin and mineral safety (these rules apply to anything you take for your health): keep them out of the reach of children, preferably in child-proof containers; and consult your doctor if you consider taking much more than the RDA for any vitamin or mineral.

While they're not dangerous, vitamins and minerals can do harm. Some of them can be toxic when taken in excess; some shouldn't be taken when you're taking certain medications; and some deplete your body of other vitamins and minerals.

Here's a look at the toxicity of the essential vitamins and minerals:

Vitamin A

If you're lost in the Arctic and starving, and somehow you manage to kill a polar bear, don't—no matter how hungry you are—eat the bear's liver. We all store Vitamin A in our liver, and polar bears store it there to an alarming degree. Too much A over a period of time can result in hair loss, nausea, headache, dry skin, bone pain, and an enlarged liver. Never take more than 25,000 I.U. daily for any length of time.

B-complex vitamins

All B-complex vitamins are essentially nontoxic, requiring absurdly high doses to do any harm (the toxic level of B_6 is 5,000 mg., while the RDA is 2 mg.). Folic acid, however, is restricted. Doses over 800 mcg. are available only through prescription, not because it's toxic (it's toxic only at higher doses) but because folic acid can mask symptoms of pernicious anemia, the B_{12} deficiency. Also of possible concern would be large doses of thiamine, which could interfere with your thyroid gland and insulin production. Large doses of niacin produce the "niacin flush," an uncomfortable but not harmful rashlike tingling that makes your complexion look red and irritated. The biggest problem with large doses of any one B vitamin is that such doses tend to deplete your other B vitamins, which is why they should all be taken together at RDA levels (they work better together).

Too much of a good thing

Remember, while too much of any good thing isn't good for you, the right amounts of these good things—vitamins and minerals—can be very good for you.

Vitamin C

Vitamin C is nontoxic, although daily doses of over 4,000 mg. (RDA is 60 mg.) can produce gas, diarrhea, dry mouth, thirst, and *maybe* kidney stones (although this last effect has been predicted, it's never been documented). High doses may also produce concentrated urine, which can be uncomfortable. The only other trouble with taking high amounts of C is that if you stop taking such doses abruptly, you may suffer from the "rebound effect"—your body becomes accustomed to the high levels and needs them to function normally. Any increase or decrease in your vitamin intake should be done slowly.

Vitamin D

High doses (over 50,000 I.U. daily; RDA is 400 I.U.) can result in decalcification—the release of calcium and phosphorus from your bones, depositing it in your blood, kidneys, heart, and lungs.

Vitamin E

Although Vitamin E is believed to cut back the cholesterol in your body, high doses (over 500 I.U. daily; RDA is 30 I.U.) may actually raise the level of triglycerides in your blood.

With this *you'll need more of* that

Some vitamins and minerals sap your body of other vitamins and minerals. So, if you're tailoring your diet toward one particular vitamin or mineral, or are taking supplements, you have to make sure you've got all your bases covered.

- *Vitamin A: Zinc depletes your Vitamin A, as does selenium. And, if you're low in A, you're probably low in C as well.*
- *B complex: Prolonged use of any one B-complex vitamin will deplete your body of other B vitamins, so it's better to take them all together (they also work better that way).*
- *Vitamin C: If you're low in C, you might also be low in A. Too much C can deplete B_{12} and folic acid.*
- *Vitamin D: Milk with synthetic Vitamin D will deplete your magnesium. Too much Vitamin D of any kind can raise your calcium levels too high.*
- *Vitamin E: Depleted by both iron and selenium.*
- *Copper: Depletes zinc.*
- *Iron: Depletes Vitamin E and is itself depleted by manganese.*
- *Magnesium: Depleted by milk with synthetic Vitamin D.*
- *Manganese: Depletes iron.*
- *Phosphorus: Depletes calcium.*
- *Potassium: Depleted by sodium.*
- *Selenium: Depletes vitamins A and E.*
- *Sodium: Depletes potassium.*
- *Zinc: Depletes Vitamin A, iron, and copper and is depleted by copper.*

Symptoms of vitamin and mineral toxicity

If you take too much of certain vitamins and minerals, they can become "poisonous," or toxic. The amount that causes toxicity varies from person to person. But when toxicity occurs, it can cause a wide variety of symptoms. Here are some of the most common:

Vitamin A
Irritability, yellow skin, hair loss, dry skin, bone and joint pain, headaches, vertigo, nausea, abdominal pain, loss of appetite.

Vitamin C
Gas, diarrhea, possible formation of urinary tract stones.

Vitamin D
Loss of appetite, nausea, vomiting, diarrhea, headache. May be followed by kidney failure and osteoporosis.

Chromium
Skin irritation and ulcers, vertigo, abdominal pain, lack of urine, shock, convulsions, coma.

Manganese
Weakness, loss of appetite, apathy, headache, impotence. May be followed by a blank face, monotone voice, tremors, rigid muscles, unusual walking patterns.

Zinc
Stomach irritation, fever, cramps, diarrhea, nausea, vomiting.

Calcium
Calcium isn't really toxic, but prolonged use of doses much more than the RDA (1,000 mg.) can lead to constipation and, possibly, kidney stones. For supplementation, use calcium gluconate or calcium carbonate. Two other common forms—bonemeal and dolomite—may contain trace amounts of lead.

Copper
You get enough copper, maybe more than enough. It's toxic in high doses, causing restlessness, insomnia, and high blood pressure. Too high levels are associated with various kinds of mental illness.

Fluorine
Fluorine is highly toxic; there's no need for supplements. You get what you need from water and toothpaste.

Iodine
Toxicity depends on your own thyroid gland—what's okay for you might be trouble for the next guy. You get enough of this if you eat seafood regularly or use iodized salt.

Iron
Children can overdose on iron (keep it out of their reach, in childproof containers). Other than that, it's nontoxic. Look for it in forms that you can use: ferr*ous*, rather than ferr*ic*.

Magnesium
Too much can have a laxative effect (epsom salts are high in magnesium, which is why people have been taking them as a laxative for years), and too high doses can bring on lethargy and drowsiness.

Manganese
When taken in very high doses, manganese can produce symptoms similar to Parkinson's disease.

Phosphorus
Phosphorus is toxic in high doses. You don't need a supplement because you get enough in your food.

Potassium
Excess potassium can produce diarrhea, irregular heartbeat, weakness, anxiety, and low blood pressure.

Medicines may change your nutritional needs

Vitamins and minerals and medicines don't always mix. In some cases, they cancel out each other's benefits. For instance, taking aspirin and Vitamin C can nullify the effects of both. In other cases, prescription and over-the-counter medicines can change your nutritional needs. If you're taking diuretics, you may need more potassium. And certain drugs, such as isoniazid and penicillamine, can increase your need for B_6.

So if you're taking medication or are receiving medical treatment, talk to your doctor about any dietary changes that you need to make.

Selenium
Although now considered essential to human health, for a long time this mineral was considered dangerous, and understandably so—it's very dangerous in large amounts. Do not exceed 500 mcg. a day.

Silicon
Sand is basically nontoxic.

Sodium
With high levels of sodium we get high blood pressure. As we get enough sodium in packaged and unpackaged food, we don't need any extra in our diet.

Zinc
Doses of 250 mg. or more (RDA is 15 mg.) can induce vomiting (doctors often use it for that very purpose), dehydration, and dizziness, among other symptoms.

Final caution
Even things like silicon that are listed as nontoxic may do harm if wolfed down by the handful. On the other hand, many of the doses mentioned would be extremely hard for you to take. For example, if one B_6 tablet contained the RDA for that vitamin, you'd have to take *2,500* of those tablets, *every day*, for *weeks* to produce a toxic reaction.

Index